Rheumatoid Arthritis

PLAN TO WIN

RHEUMATOID ARTHRITIS

PLAN TO WIN

Cheryl Koehn
Taysha Palmer
John Esdaile, M.D.

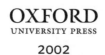

OXFORD
UNIVERSITY PRESS

2002

OXFORD
UNIVERSITY PRESS

Oxford New York

Athens Auckland Bangkok Bogotá Buenos Aires Cape Town
Chennai Dar es Salaam Delhi Florence Hong Kong Istanbul Karachi
Kolkata Kuala Lumpur Madrid Melbourne Mexico City Mumbai Nairobi
Paris São Paulo Shanghai Singapore Taipei Tokyo Toronto Warsaw

and associated companies in

Berlin Ibadan

Published by Oxford University Press, Inc.
198 Madison Avenue, New York, New York, 10016
http://www.oup-usa.org

Oxford is a registered trademark of Oxford University Press

Library of Congress Cataloging-in-Publication Data
Koehn, Cheryl.
   Rheumatoid arthritis : plan to win / Cheryl Koehn, Taysha Palmer, John Esdaile.
     p. cm.
   ISBN 0-19-513056-1 (cloth)
   1. Rheumatoid arthritis—Popular works. I. Palmer, Taysha. II. Esdaile, John. III. Title.

RC933. .K64 2001
616.7'227—dc21   2001032165

Dose schedules are being continually revised and new side effects recognized.
Research into other aspects of health care and wellness are also ongoing.
Oxford University Press and the authors make no representation,
express or implied, that the medications and dosages outlined in this book
are correct. For these reasons, readers are strongly urged to consult their physicians
and the pharmaceutical company's printed instructions before taking any medications,
and also before undertaking exercise programs or following other recommendations
made in this book.

Book design and composition by Susan Day.

9 8 7 6 5 4 3 2 1
Printed in the United States of America
on acid-free paper

Contents

This book is a fine pearl. I will recommend it to my patients, their families, and to their health care providers. It is the only book about rheumatoid arthritis written by a person with it, a physician, and a medical writer. As such, it is a poignant, understandable, calm guide for what to expect and how to prevail.

Life deals a hard hand to some individuals, which they neither deserve, nor in many instances can control. For most people with rheumatoid arthritis, it is a lifelong journey and, I believe, an experience that brings special insights about oneself, what is important in life, and draws out and on all of one's inner resources.

I first met Ms. Koehn at a landmark meeting organized by The Arthritis Society in the shadow of the Canadian Parliament. It was the first attempt to bring together the many persons and organizations concerned with these disorders, but it became a forum for lament and blame. That all changed when Ms. Koehn, who was in the audience, stood up and gave an impassioned plea that changed the course of the meeting and, as history subsequently showed, the course of Canadian rheumatologic care. I suspect this book will have the same kind of positive impact on individuals with rheumatoid arthritis. It is a comprehensive and thoroughly researched book that will help patients, their families, and their providers to negotiate the vagaries of a waxing waning illness in which the issues of the moment need to be solved with a view to the future.

There are many self-help books, but there are none that deal realistically, accurately, and emotionally with the many issues that confront the person with RA. The result—this gem—is the gist of a conversation between a special, wise physician who is an expert about what's known and not known; a professional medical writer, a master at making technical material accessible to others; and a woman who has lived a decade with a chronic and (for now) incurable illness who lives a full life as a person, not a victim, not a patient. As a "survivor," she knows more about what matters most to people with rheumatoid arthritis than most anyone I have found or worked with, and I might add, myself.

Matthew H. Liang, M.D., M.P.H.
Professor of Medicine, Harvard Medical School
Professor of Health Policy and Management,
    Harvard School of Public Health
Director, Robert B. Brigham Arthritis and Musculoskeletal
    Clinical Research Center

Acknowledgments

There are so many people to thank; so many friends to acknowledge.

First and foremost, thanks to our editor at Oxford University Press, Joan Bossert. Without her belief, guidance, expertise, and patience, this book truly would not exist.

For able research assistance, we'd like to acknowledge Jolanda Cibere, Sharon Demeter, Misti Farrish, Allen Lehman, Helen Langford, Diane Lacaille, Jean Lederer, Sherrie Lynch, Sheri MacIntyre and Cheryl Pinto. For artistic contributions, much appreciation goes to John Marsala and Sue Smith.

For professional review and input, we give many thanks to physiotherapist Bruce Clark, occupational therapist Lori Cyr, nurse midwife Sharon Demeter, rheumatologist Bob Offer, nurse Susan Offer, social worker Greg Taylor, and nurse Karen Rangno. We also thank Gideon Koren, director and head of the MotherRisk Program, who provided constructive comments on medication use in pregnancy and breastfeeding.

We offer boundless gratitude to colleagues, friends, family, and people living with RA who shared their expertise, support, enthusiasm and patience during the writing of this book. In particular, our appreciation goes to Tim Boychuk, Bev Holmes, John Hurst, Alice Klinkhoff, Bill Langlois, Ricki Lambeck-McConchie, Denis Morrice, Kevin Noel, Sue Paine and Don Sancton and Pfizer Canada, whose early support was instrumental in getting this book off the ground.

Special thanks to Sharon Demeter, for the wisdom inherent in the special message to partners of people with RA; and to Matt Liang, our friend, colleague, and walking repository of all things good, for writing the book's foreword.

THRIVING WITH RA

*A message from Cheryl Koehn,
coauthor of* PLAN TO WIN *and person with RA*

What lies behind you, what lies ahead of you,
pales in comparison to what lies within you.

—Ralph Waldo Emerson

It may sound strange—especially if you're newly or recently diagnosed—but having RA these past ten years has been an inspiring and rewarding experience for me. You may think I'm foolish, possibly even heartless, to promote the notion of thriving with RA, but I know that's what I've done—and I know you can too.

You see, I've been where you are: in pain, frightened, confused, and feeling alone. I know there are days ahead of me when I'll be there once again, for that's the nature of the RA beast. What comforts me and gives me confidence to live each day to the fullest is that I have a PLAN TO WIN. I have learned as much as I can about RA and have an excellent team of family, friends, and health care professionals to call on when I need help. I make informed choices about every aspect of my treatment plan. I am in control of all that I can control, and you can be, too.

It wasn't always that way. When I woke up mornings during the early going of my disease I had to soak my feet in buckets of ice water to ease the pain and swelling to walk. My fingers were so inflamed and stiff I couldn't brush my hair or teeth. When my knees and shoulders were hot and painful and I could not sleep, I can honestly say that I thought the rest of my life would be filled with misery. Thankfully, I was wrong.

What I learned in my first year living with RA was that with a solid plan in place—a plan that included an expert health care team, early aggressive medication therapy, exercise, and counseling, among other things—I could do most of the things I did before I got RA, some, a whole lot better.

The things I do include listening to my body and treating it with kindness; communicating my needs to family, friends and coworkers; leading my health care team; finding meaning in my work and life; and taking care of the inner "CK."

With my own PLAN TO WIN, I run my marketing communications consulting business, rollerblade and ski (with care!), work out at the gym (with care!), advocate for more and better arthritis research, treatment, and education, and be in incredible loving relationships with my husband, family, and friends. I know you, too, can have a rich and rewarding life with RA.

Be well, and PLAN TO WIN!

Cheryl Koehn

Rheumatoid Arthritis

PLAN TO WIN

That is not to say you won't face challenges along the way—challenges that for many seem insurmountable. Early on, there will be days when simply thinking about your RA wrenches your heart and soul. Days when you are angry that it "happened to you." Days when you feel as though no one understands—or cares—what it is you are going through. Days when you fear what RA will do next.

When you face these darker days—and you most certainly will—just know that you are not alone. An abundance of resources exist to help you learn to live with the disease in the most healthful way possible—there's information on these throughout the PLAN TO WIN.

The PLAN TO WIN contains nine basic principles or guidelines—principles that have been proven to help people with RA and other chronic conditions claim back their lives from the disease, and enjoy optimal health.

P   Plan for my return to optimal health
L   Learn to get the most from my health care team
A   Accept personal responsibility for things I can control
N   Notice and record changes in my mind and body

T   Take charge of my treatment plan
O   Optimize my environment and energy use

W   Work toward healthy relationships with self and others
I   Integrate healthy eating, exercise, and mind-body awareness
N   Never give in to RA

The information in this book supports the PLAN TO WIN, and serves as your own personal RA expert, one who is available twenty-four hours a day, seven days a week, 365 days a year. Your expert provides the most up-to-date information on research and treatments and acts as a reliable companion for emotional support and practical tips.

As you learn about RA over time and gain experience with how it is affecting your body, you will become expert at living with the disease. Sharing your expertise with your physicians and other health care professionals will be instrumental in getting you all working as a team to gain control over the disease. Also, learning to understand what's going on inside your mind and heart, and sharing this information with those closest to you will be essential in managing the change that occurs in relationships when dealing with a health challenge such as RA.

Of course, no PLAN TO WIN would be complete without incorporating a guideline for overall health—integration of healthy eating, exercise, emotional wellness, and *a positive attitude.*

Taking care of the whole "you" is a key aspect of the PLAN TO WIN. Eating

Chapter 1

PLAN TO WIN

"If you think you can win, you can win. Faith is necessary to victory."

—William Hazlitt

Every day, people make plans—for small things like seeing a movie with a friend or running errands around town, to realizing larger life goals such as attending college or pursuing a career change. We plan vacations, finances—even our gardens are planned.

Successful people everywhere take that planning one step further. They take great care in thinking through the things they most want to have or accomplish in life, then making plans to accomplish those goals and "working" their plans until their dreams are realized.

For you, and the nearly 2.5 million others in North America diagnosed with rheumatoid arthritis (RA), developing a solid plan and seeing it through is essential to realizing one of the most valuable goals *anyone* can attain in life—enjoyment of optimal health.

In the PLAN TO WIN, we do not propose a miracle cure or an "easy way out" of having RA. This book is about a plan to minimize, possibly even beat, the potentially devastating effects of RA in your life.

What we have done is assemble the scientific knowledge gained from thousands of research studies around the world, involving people of all ages and severity of disease. We have used the findings from these studies to create a blueprint called the PLAN TO WIN. Of course, the PLAN TO WIN is merely that: a blueprint. Together with health professionals expert in arthritis, you will help pour the foundation; construct a solid frame; and put on the finishing touches that will make this plan your own. By using the information in this book as a starting point, you will be better able to make well-informed decisions about your treatment plan, and you'll stand an excellent chance of living a fulfilling, productive life with RA.

to energize and maintain nutrient levels in your body, exercising to build or regain strength to support your joint and skeletal system, and focusing on "winning" will move you forward faster toward optimal health.

THE PLAN TO WIN

Planning for Your Return to Optimal Health

Having a plan to win means determining what it is that you want—in your case, optimal health—and taking action to get it. Educate yourself about all aspects of RA: understanding it, living with it, and making decisions to control it.

Identify what steps you want to take to gain back optimal health, and prioritize which ones you will take first. Establish a start date for each step, and, where applicable, a completion date—some steps will be ongoing, such as taking medication, exercising, and eating healthfully.

When you make decisions regarding your health care, be responsible for them and ensure those decisions are carried out (either by yourself or another). Doing so will put you in control and leave you feeling good at the end of each day.

Make a personal contract with yourself to follow the PLAN TO WIN and tape it to your clothes closet door or bathroom mirror to remind you of your commitment to the plan—and to yourself.

Learning to Get the Most From Your Health Care Team

During the early days following diagnosis, you may encounter major forces to reckon with, such as: pain more intense than you ever imagined possible; inflammation or swelling in your joints, restricted ability to move (which may mean loss of the ability to work, lift your children, or even shop for groceries), and the deep fear that can accompany all of these changes. But just as you might do when strategizing to win a tennis match or land an important deal, learn all that you can about RA and use effective response measures that help you win.

Working with a team of arthritis experts will help you manage the disease rather than letting it manage you. Your team of experts might include a rheumatologist (a doctor who specializes in arthritis and related diseases); a physical therapist (who helps with pain and movement problems); an occupational therapist (who can teach you ways to protect joints, conserve energy, and still get things done); a counselor (who can assist with emotional and relationship issues); and others as you identify a need. With you as "captain," these individuals make up your health care "team."

Learn to work with your team, as well as to rely on them as you may need to throughout the course of your disease. Accept that while you're the leader of the team, some days will be more challenging than others and may require you to "lean" rather than lead.

Accepting Personal Responsibility for Things You Can Control

By following the PLAN TO WIN, you will automatically begin taking responsibility for factors within your control: factors such as communicating to your health care team how your body feels in response to their prescribed treatments; adhering to medication schedules and dietary plans; exercising safely and regularly; and so on. Remember, while you are in the best position to be in charge of your treatment plan, you will rely on the experienced and dedicated professionals on your health care team every step of the way.

Noticing and Recording Health Changes

As you live with RA, you will learn to manage the "ebb and flow" nature of the disease. Monitoring and evaluating your progress on a regular basis is one sure way to keep track of how you are doing. (This is especially true when making decisions about medication.)

Regularly collect information on all aspects of your treatment plan in a journal and share it with all of the members of your health care team. If there are aspects of your plan that aren't producing the results you expected as quickly as you expected them, discuss your concerns with the other members of your team and consider modifying your plan. As a team, explore and discuss alternate or additional treatment options and, before making a decision, carefully weigh the benefits and risks of each option before making a change.

Taking Charge of Your Treatment Plan

While arthritis researchers are dogged in their pursuit of the cause(s) of RA and an eventual cure, people living with the disease today require therapies that effectively manage and control both symptoms and the disease. By knowing all that you can about RA; developing the skills to build and lead an expert health care team; recognizing the short- and long-term benefits of initiating early treatment and understanding the difference between proven and unproven therapies; exploring the relationship between mind and body; you will have the ability to take charge of your treatment plan by making informed decisions.

The goal is to become the expert on *your* disease—the disease course and response to therapy is different in each individual. By developing this expertise, you are well equipped to know what works to keep symptoms under control, and whether your treatment goals are being met. Ask questions if you're not sure. You have a right to know everything you can about your treatment options and your RA.

Optimizing Your Environment and Energy Use

Living day-to-day with RA can be challenging at the best of times, but optimizing one's physical environment and managing energy use can be indispensable to maintaining quality of life.

There are myriad ways to modify your physical environments at home and work, allowing you to do the things you need and want to do. There are a growing number of "arthritis friendly" products (e.g., cooking and gardening implements, office furniture, lighting, etc.) available today, as well as funding from nonprofit and government agencies to assist with major modifications you may need to make to your home and place of work. Take full advantage of these resources (where and when needed) to make your environment easier to live and work in.

Optimize energy by knowing how much of it you have and by prioritizing how you spend it. Call on family members or friends to assist with tasks and daily activities you find difficult to handle, and schedule those that require more energy for periods in the day or week when you are well rested and experiencing the least amount of pain and stiffness.

When ready, speak to your employer and let him/her know about your diagnosis. Together, you can look for ways to manage tasks or responsibilities that are difficult given your disease. Whether the solution is to work less during periods of greater disease activity, to job share, or to shift or exchange present responsibilities for ones that are more "RA friendly," a solution can be found.

Working Toward Healthy Relationships with Self and Others

The pain and physical limitations RA imposes can have a direct effect on you and those in your life. At times, it can seem that living with RA is equivalent to riding on a roller coaster, with emotions going up and down alongside that of the disease's activity.

To disembark the RA roller coaster, develop a network of friends and family with whom you can share your feelings, and consider seeking professional counseling for problems that may seem overwhelming and leave you feeling helpless. Welcome opportunities to explore what's going on inside your head and your heart, and courageously share your feelings with people you trust and respect.

Integrating Healthy Eating, Exercise, and Mind-Body Awareness

Healthy living means embracing lifestyle habits that contribute to a sense of wellness and normality: healthy eating, exercise, and mind-body awareness.

Most know that regular exercise will strengthen the body and help to maintain ideal body weight. But what you really need to know is that regular exercise (for flexibility, strengthening, and a cardiovascular workout) will help your body deal with the specific challenges of RA—inflammation, stiffness, and pain. And along with the physical benefits exercise delivers come the psychological "perks"—increases in self-confidence and self-esteem.

For the person with RA, eating healthfully requires knowledge and planning. The disease itself can rob the body of nutrients that are vital for the body to grow new tissue and bone, and several of the medication therapies tend to throw off the body's delicate nutritional balance. As such, you will want to pay extra attention to how you "fuel" your body with food. The right mixes of vitamins and minerals, dietary starch, fiber, protein, and oils will help keep your body on an even nutritional keel while winning against RA.

Mind-body awareness plays a fundamental role in winning, too. It can boost your immune, hormonal, and cardiovascular systems; help control pain and inflammation; and actually increase the likelihood you will get helpful support as well as take the necessary steps to exercise and eat well.

Never give in to RA

When facing illness or adversity, there are times when it can be tempting to give in and stop trying. It's at these times you will have to dig deep and tap into your inner strength, which will be necessary to keep moving you forward. Look in the mirror and tell yourself, I can do it—I can win. If your body hurts and you're having difficulties managing even the simplest tasks at home or work, tell yourself—out loud—I'm doing great, I'm getting better. *Make a commitment to yourself to never give in to RA.*

AND NOW ... ON TO WINNING!

Each of the chapters in this book contain information from the most reliable studies and arthritis health professionals around the world. What you will find in the following chapters, organized by topic, is information you can rely on when carrying out your own personal PLAN TO WIN.

Step one in winning against RA is filling your knowledge bank with information about the disease itself. In Chapter 2, we tell you what the words "rheumatoid arthritis" mean, who gets the disease and at what age, how to recognize RA symptoms, how joints and internal organs may be affected, about the possible causes of RA, and much more.

Chapter 3 describes why building an experienced RA health care team is important, how to build the team, about the services each team member provides, and how to communicate and work with team members to ensure you get the most—and best—of what they have to offer.

Chapter 4 provides an in-depth look at RA medications, the reasons behind employing their use early on, combination therapy, keeping track of how you feel when taking RA medications, strategies for dealing with concern about side effects and for staying on medication regimes, detailed descriptions of each medication, emerging therapies, and experimental therapies.

Chapter 5 and Chapter 6 detail how exercise, diet, and nutrition can help your body survive the short- and long-term effects of RA, and include easy-to-reference exercise diagrams and descriptions, as well as tips on healthy living and eating.

Chapter 7 explores the emotional and psychological aspects of living with RA, and explains the research that's been done on how RA affects the individual living with the disease and those around them. It describes eight attitudes and attributes that support health, and suggests practices that can enhance mind-body awareness.

Chapter 8, gives detailed information on how RA can affect your relationships at work and home, describes helpful and unhelpful support, provides useful communication tips, and offers practical advice on maintaining a healthy and satisfying sexual life with RA. This chapter also includes a special "Message to Spouses and Partners."

Chapter 9 is filled with practical information on living day-to-day with RA. From help with identifying problems and creating solutions to advice on adapting daily tasks and joint protection, this chapter is a "must read" for gaining back and maintaining quality of life.

Understanding the role of surgery in managing long-term RA is another important aspect of maintaining quality of life. Chapter 10 explores the types of surgery available to people with RA today, offers advice on how to decide when the time is right, and gives tips on preparing for, and recovering from, surgery.

Chapter 11 provides in-depth pregnancy information not found in other books on RA. It disscusses the remission from RA that pregnancy often affords, as well as the chances of postpregnancy disease activity; gives information on maximizing your liklihood of having a healthy pregnancy and childbirth, provides a detailed chart of RA medications and their use (or restriction) before and during pregnancy and while breast-feeding; and offers strategies for making baby care easier if or when a postchildbirth flare strikes.

Recognizing that you'll want to learn more as you live with RA, Chapter 12 offers you myriad places to look for reliable information about the disease and its management.

Chapter 2

THE FACTS ABOUT
RHEUMATOID ARTHRITIS (RA)

"Education, c'est delivrance."
("Education is freedom.")

—André Gide

The PLAN TO WIN begins with arming yourself with knowledge about RA. Understanding what a diagnosis of RA means, recognizing symptoms, knowing how they affect your joints and internal organs, and exploring the causes of RA, all provide you with the information you need to make sense of what is happening in your body.

Knowing these facts will enable you to have informed discussions with your rheumatologist (a physician specializing in arthritis detection and treatment) and other members of your health care team, and help you make sound decisions about all aspects of your treatment plan. By learning as much as possible about RA, you can gain a sense of control over the disease, and ultimately, achieve optimal health.

It may take several readings of this chapter before you understand the complexities of the cause and course of RA. You may wish to make notes as you read along, then ask your physician for clarification, if necessary.

SYMPTOMS AND SIGNS OF RA

For one person in three, RA starts suddenly over several days or over as long as several weeks. For most (the remaining two out of three), it starts more gradually over a period of several weeks to several months. In about 5 percent of people with RA, the disease will disappear over a period of four to eight weeks after it starts. For another 10 percent, there may be temporary periods of improvement that, on rare occasions, last several years. For the majority of people (85 percent), RA is a chronic (ongoing) disease in which they may have periods of comparative improvement. But untreated or even ineffectively treated, over the long run, the disease progresses with increasing damage and increasing limitation on being able to do the things one wants to in life.

RA is a system-wide disease. It is not confined to the joints but can affect much of the body. The first symptoms and signs usually appear in the joints. "Symptoms" are things you feel or experience that your physician can't see, and "signs" are things your physician (usually a rheumatologist) can observe. The first symptoms are of joint stiffness and joint pain—this is what you feel. The first sign is joint swelling. This is what both you and your doctor can observe. The affected joints are almost always stiff and painful. What is a vague pain one day may be more persistent and associated with obvious swelling of the joint within weeks. Along with the joint stiffness, joint pain, and joint swelling, another symptom, fatigue, is often present. Joint stiffness, joint pain, fatigue, and joint swelling are the hallmark symptoms and signs of RA.

Inflammation

The cause of these symptoms and signs of RA is inflammation. The word "inflammation" means something has been literally "set on fire." The severe pain of a strep throat infection is an example of inflammation that most of us have experienced. The pain is unrelenting; swallowing becomes very painful. In RA, it is the joints that have been set on fire—a great many of them, and this explains the joint swelling, stiffness, pain, and, also, the fatigue. Inflammation of the joints is called *synovitis.*

Detecting the mild warmth that may be present early on is not always easy. It is usually most noticeable in large joints that are close to the skin, such as the knee and the ankle. While not as essential a feature as joint stiffness, joint pain, or joint swelling, joint warmth helps rheumatologists confirm a diagnosis of RA.

The healthy joint contains a membrane or lining called the *synovium* (Figure 2.1). The lining normally is thin—only a few cells thick—like a sheet of newspaper. It makes and maintains a small amount of fluid required for the joint's proper functioning. The fluid nourishes the joint and acts as a lubricant during joint movement. In RA, this lining is inflamed. It is thickened and appears angry red. This inflamed lining makes extra joint fluid. Thus, the joint becomes swollen, both because the lining is inflamed and thickened, and because the inflamed lining is making extra fluid.

As a result, your knuckles are hard to see when you make a fist, rings are difficult to get off, knees appear bigger, and shoes that were once comfortable become tight and painful. In RA, many joints are usually swollen. Early on, when the inflammation is just starting, the swelling may be subtle and you may not notice the full extent of it. It can take the skill of a rheumatol-

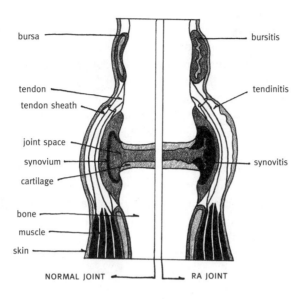

Fig. 2.1. Normal joint on the left and RA joint on the right. The synovium is a thin lining that makes the fluid that is present in small amounts in a normal joint. The fluid nourishes the joint and lubricates it. In RA, the inflammation of the lining thickens it, more fluid is made, and the joint swells as a result. The inflamed lining can damage the cartilage and nearby bone by releasing inflammatory substances and by direct attack. The lining of tendons is similar to the lining of the joint. It can become inflamed in RA. Finally, a bursa is literally a small sac that normally protects a tendon or joint. A bursa also has a lining that can become inflamed, resulting in extra fluid production and swelling.

ogist to make a correct diagnosis promptly. Swollen joints are a key feature of RA, and their detection is crucial to timely diagnosis of the disease.

Tendon sheaths are similar to joint lining (Figure 2.1). They line the tendon like a shirt sleeve lines an arm. Tendon sheaths are often involved in RA and when affected can damage the tendons that are needed to make a joint move. When the tendon itself is inflamed, it is called *tendinitis*, and when tendon sheaths are inflamed, it is called *tenosynovitis*. Tendon sheaths all over the body may be affected in RA. However, those responsible for moving the fingers at the wrist are involved most commonly and can cause pressure on nerves, tendon damage, and even tendon breakage.

Many joints have protective sacs or *bursa* to protect them from friction from tendons and muscles as well as from external pressure. Bursa are lined by a tissue similar to joint lining. Like joints and tendon sheaths, bursa can become inflamed. Inflammation of a bursa, called *bursitis*, can also cause damage, especially in the neck, where it results in the loosening of the vertebrae high in the neck. Other common sites for bursitis in RA are the shoulder, the elbow, the hip, and the knee. Tendinitis, tenosynovitis, and bursitis all add to the stiffness and pain of RA.

ˌS

med joint becomes stiff when it is not used. The longest period of ˌest comes with sleep, so joint stiffness, or what doctors call "early morning stiffness," is present the moment one awakens in the morning. However, stiffness or "gelling" also can occur after briefer periods of rest, such as sitting for a meal or going for a car ride. Most people have experienced joint stiffness at some time—after a prolonged ride in a cramped car seat, for example. Usually, after a minute or two of walking, the joints move normally again. But in RA, the stiffness that results from inactivity is prolonged and severe. It may last for more than an hour after you get up in the morning. The worse the inflammation, the longer the early morning stiffness or gelling. When the disease is acting up (often called a "flare"), early morning stiffness will last several hours or even all day. Also, RA joint stiffness is much more severe than the few minutes' stiffness the healthy person feels on climbing out of a car. At its worst, the stiffness can limit your ability to perform everyday activities, such as eating, dressing, walking, or working.

Pain

It is the rare person who has not sprained an ankle or twisted a knee and had to limp around for several days, perhaps receiving sympathy from family, friends, and coworkers. For a person with RA, the pain is at least this intense, but twenty, thirty, or even more joints are painful—all the time. The sprained ankle or twisted knee feels better when we elevate it. By contrast, prolonged resting makes RA pain worse. When the RA inflammation is poorly controlled, you may not only have pain all day but also awaken nightly with severe joint pain. Joint pain due to inflammation may actually improve a little when the joints are moved about a bit. However, sleeping pills do nothing to prevent the severe pain during the night and painkillers do little. Only therapy directed at limiting the RA inflammation really helps (more on this later). Joint pain is another key feature of RA.

Fatigue

Fatigue is another constant reminder of RA. The extra joint fluid in RA is not an excess amount of normal fluid. It is an inflammatory soup, filled with inflammatory cells that, along with the joint lining cells, release chemicals that actually cause the joint stiffness and the joint pain. The inflammatory chemicals do not remain confined to the joints but spill over into the rest of your body. Early on, fatigue is the main complaint that results from these inflammatory substances outside the joint. Having active RA is like having a severe cold or flu. But instead of the fatigue improving after several days as it would with the flu, it persists. It is unrelenting. If you are an active individual who has always been able to go all day, you may suddenly need a nap every afternoon.

WHO GETS RA

About 0.5 percent to 1.0 percent (1 in 200 to 1 in 100) of the population have RA. Two or three women are affected for every man with the disease. The frequency of RA varies based on ethnic background. Only 0.1 percent of native Africans develop RA, but up to 5 percent of Native North Americans get the disease. Otherwise, there does not appear to be any difference in the frequency of RA based on how far north or south you live or whether the climate is dry or wet, hot or cold.

As people become older, their chance of developing RA grows a little higher each year, at least until they are in their sixties and seventies. Thus, the frequency of *new* cases of RA keeps increasing with age. For example, in a given year, more new cases of RA develop in people aged 51 to 60 than develop among an identical number of people aged 41 to 50.

It is interesting that RA may be a "new" disease in Europeans. It was first described in the medical literature in 1800, and conditions similar to RA are depicted in European paintings as far back as the mid-fifteenth century. In contrast, RA has been identified in Native American skeletons in the Mississippi River valley as far back as 4500 BC. Some have suggested that RA originated as an infection among a small group of Native Americans and subsequently spread worldwide.

THE CAUSE OF RA

We do not know what causes RA, but that is not to say nothing is known. The past two decades have seen an unprecedented advance in our knowledge of RA. (In later chapters, we will discuss the impact this increase in knowledge has had on treatment.) We have learned that RA is a disease of great complexity. We do not know the cause or the exact mechanisms that perpetuate the RA process, but researchers are making progress on several theories.

Theory 1: Infection as a Cause

Infection as a cause of RA is not a new idea, but so far, scientists have not proven the theory. In 1900, the eminent international physician, Sir William Osler, believed that infection, particularly dental infection, was the cause of RA. This led to unnecessary removal of many teeth but no reduction or amelioration in RA. The suggestion that RA started in the Mississippi River valley and spread around the world from there also raises the possibility of the disease having been spread through infection.

When bacteria gain direct access to a joint cavity, this is called *infectious arthritis*. This has an abrupt onset and promptly results in severe joint damage. It is a medical emergency. Usually only one joint is infected and the suddenness of the onset makes it distinguishable from RA. However, other bacteria can enter the body and trigger an arthritis without actually infecting the joints. Some of these types of arthritis resemble RA. Rheumatic fever, a condition caused by the body's immune reaction to certain streptococcal bacteria, results in arthritis. However, the arthritis of rheumatic fever does not cause permanent joint damage, as does RA. Lyme disease, which was called Lyme arthritis before it was recognized to involve other organs, is caused by a bacteria and can cause permanent joint damage, at least in some people. Certain other bacteria—such as shigella, salmonella, campylobacter, and chlamydia—can cause diarrhea or infection of the genitourinary (kidney and bladder) system. In some, but not all, individuals with just the right genetic makeup, these bacteria can trigger a chronic damaging arthritis. Again, in these types of arthritis, the bacteria are not causing the disease directly, as they do with a tooth abscess or a strep throat. The bacteria trigger a response in the body that causes the arthritis, essentially by mistake. Not only bacteria, but also viruses, such as rubella (German measles) and parvovirus, can trigger an arthritis, although usually permanent damage does not result.

Yet, despite intensive research using the most sophisticated techniques available, an infectious cause for *rheumatoid* arthritis has not been identified. It seems likely that if infection is involved in the cause of RA, it is only part of the cause. Or, perhaps, a number of different infections may have the ability to cause RA, and depending on genetic makeup, may initiate the disease in one person—but not in the next.

Theory 2: The Role of Genes in RA

For a long time, scientists have believed that genes play a role in RA. It is known that if one member of a family has RA, another family member is three or four times more likely to develop RA than one would expect. This suggests a genetic component, as each child receives half their genes from their mother and half from their father. Thus, sisters and brothers share a lot of genes. The three or four fold increase in the frequency of RA among people who share genes (that is, family members) when one person in the family has RA, compared to families with no one with RA, could be due to a common gene. However, because children grow up together, the RA also could be caused by a similar exposure in childhood, such as infection.

Additional information on the importance of genes comes from the study of twins. If one twin develops RA, the second is more likely to develop RA if they are identical twins than if they are nonidentical twins. Identical twins are genetically identical, rather like carbon copies. Nonidentical twins are like ordinary brothers and sisters. They are about 50 percent identical. If RA was caused *only* by something in the environment, like an infection, a food, or a chemical, then one would expect identical and nonidentical twins to be equally as likely to "catch" RA. However, the higher frequency of RA in identical twins compared to nonidentical twins means that genes must play a role in the cause of RA.

The *human leucocyte antigen* (HLA) has been shown to play a key role in the human body's ability to reject a kidney, a heart, or some other transplanted organ. This knowledge was essential to the great strides that have been made in transplanting organs from one human to another. Advance in one area of science often has spinoffs in others, and this was the case with HLA. It was soon recognized that a specific HLA gene marker, called HLA-DRB1, was present in RA more often than would be expected. Subsequent research showed the association with RA is confined to a tiny portion of the HLA-DRB1 gene—specifically amino acid proteins number 67 to 74 (amino acids are the building blocks that make up a protein). The sequence forms a small docking station in the molecule. A disproportionately high frequency of the same docking station is found in genes of persons with RA, regardless of their ethnic origin. This is new and very promising research.

Although the way the RA docking station interacts as part of the RA process is not yet known, there are several possible explanations. One is that the docking station could interact with the substance that actually causes RA. If correct, a specific agent, such as an infectious agent, would literally enter the docking station and lock on, thereby causing RA. Understandably, scientists are investigating what could enter the docking station. Second, we know the HLA region plays an important role in the success of kidney, heart, and other organ transplants and oversees the body's defense against all things foreign (such as someone else's kidney or a bacteria). It controls the immune defense system, guiding the attack on bacteria, viruses, foreign tissues such as transplants, and even cancer cells. It is thought the specific RA docking station may influence the immune cells that are known to be essential to keeping the RA process going. Thus, a process that would normally have stopped is encouraged to continue. Third, the protein docking station could itself be mistaken by the immune system as something unacceptable or foreign (perhaps an infectious agent). In this case, the body's immune system would start an attack against its own tissues, thinking it was protecting itself from foreign attack.

As exciting and important as the information on the HLA-DRB1 gene is, scientists know it is not the complete story. The HLA-DRB1 gene is linked to disease progression and prognosis (a commonly used medical word that means how the person will do). Those with more severe RA are more likely to have the HLA-DRB1 marker, making scientists believe that it plays a role in determining how a person who has developed RA will do, over time, rather than actually causing the disease. More research is clearly needed, but it is now thought that there are multiple RA genes. The exact number is not known. Some of the RA genes may be important in allowing the disease to start, while others cause it to continue. But, even if a person had all the genes needed to cause RA, they still might not develop the disease. In some individuals, the genes will depend on yet other factors for their action (e.g., factors relating to ethnicity have been suggested as important) or they may need to interact with one or more different inciting agents, those as yet elusive infectious or chemical triggers.

We have learned that the genetics of RA are complex, so the hunt for the RA genes is extremely challenging and is the forefront of current RA research. To identify the RA genes, American investigators and colleagues around the world are collaborating in assembling one thousand families in which multiple family members have RA. New techniques that did not exist even a few years ago will be used to identify the RA genes. Once the genes have been identified, understanding what the genes do individually, how they act in concert, and determining which of the actions result in RA will be even harder than the identification of the genes.

RA has proven a complicated foe for scientists. Nonetheless, more and more is being learned each day and the pace is gaining speed. Nowhere has the progress been greater than in our understanding of the RA disease process itself. As will be discussed in Chapter 4, some of this knowledge is already being translated into effective treatments.

THE RA ATTACK INSIDE THE JOINT

The cause of RA may be elusive, but the progress in our understanding of the disease process *after* RA begins has been significant—and has led to better treatment. After RA starts, its major attack is on the lining of the joint, or synovium. As mentioned earlier, in RA, the synovium thickens due to inflammation. The cells that form the normal joint lining become harmful rather than beneficial. With time, the inflamed lining tissues invade and damage the nearby *cartilage* (cartilage is the gristle that is the smooth surface covering the end of the bone in a normal joint) and the underlying bone (Figure 2.1).

As part of these changes, the joint's lining attracts *white blood cells* from the bloodstream. White blood cells are defense cells that rid the body of infection and other things that should not be there. In addition to destroying bacteria, viruses, and other foreign agents that may enter the body, the white blood cells have other roles. For example, when you get a cut that becomes infected, white blood cells lead the cleanup of this debris created by the battle to eliminate that infection, and they are involved in the repair of the cut. They also act as memory cells, so if a bacteria or virus gains entry again, the response will be even swifter.

There are a number of different families of white blood cells. The *poly* (short for polymorphonuclear white blood cell) family can ingest bacteria and liquefy them with potent destructive enzymes. The joint lining and the extra fluid that is present in the RA joint are loaded with polys, even though there are no bacteria or foreign agents present. Nonetheless, they release their harmful enzymes. The ability of the poly to create molecules called *prostaglandins* is the basis of using nonsteroidal anti-inflammatory drugs (called NSAIDS for short, including aspirin, ibuprofen, naproxen, diclofenac, and, increasingly, celecoxib and rofecoxib), to treat against inflammation and pain. The NSAIDS inhibit the production of the prostaglandins and diminish the pain associated with RA.

Another family of white blood cells is the *monocyte/macrophage* group. While the poly is the expert at grabbing and destroying bacteria, the monocytes and macrophage cells collect the debris after battle—the body's garbage collectors. They also recognize when something is foreign. When they do detect an intruder or foreign protein, they take action to alert the other cells in the body's defense system, and are important in developing the memory cells that will guard against renewed invasion.

Considerable recent attention has focused on a third family known as the *lymphocytes*. It has become apparent these play a vital role in the body's defense (or immune) system. There are two branches to the lymphocyte family: B and T. The *B lymphocytes* make our *antibodies* (proteins that protect us against infection). For instance, a polio vaccine or a tetanus shot results in the body making protective antibodies against polio virus and tetanus toxin, respectively. A single B cell will make an antibody against only one thing—a B cell making antibodies against polio would not make them against tetanus toxin. It turns out that many of the antibody-making cells in the joint lining of a person with RA are making *rheumatoid factor*, the antibody that is detected in the RA blood test. From blood tests in people with RA, we know that the more rheumatoid factor antibody present in the blood, the more severe the RA tends to be. This led to the belief that the rheumatoid factor or RA antibody was a harmful antibody—that it participated directly in the RA damage. However, some scientists now believe that the rheumatoid factor antibody is formed as part of an attempt by the body to limit the damage. Whichever is correct, the inflamed joint lining contains many cells that are making rheumatoid factor, so even though it may be uncertain whether rheumatoid factor is a harmful or a protective antibody, it must be important to what is going on.

The other branch of this white blood cell family are the T lymphocytes. There are a number of different categories of *T lymphocyte*. The one that is the most common in the inflamed RA joint lining is called the CD4 T cell. The exact role of the CD4 T cell is unresolved, but is attracting considerable research interest. It is thought that the types of CD4 cells available in RA are faulty and skewed toward an overabundance of CD4 cells that are *autode-*

structive—that is, they target the normal body tissues rather than foreign agents, such as bacteria. Not only is there an increase in cells that can lead an attack on normal tissue, but there also is a decrease in the type of T cells that play a protective role. Out-of-control destructive CD4 T cells appear to be important in the progression of RA.

The CD4 T cell interacts with other synovial cells, including the monocyte/macrophage white blood cells. The T cell is capable of making *cytokines*—molecules that can act as messengers to magnify or diminish the inflammatory attack. The monocytes, including those in the joint lining, also produce cytokines. Two of these cytokines have become important targets for new treatments. They are *IL-1* (IL stands for interleukin) and *TNF-alpha* (TNF stands for tumor necrosis factor; the first function identified for TNF by scientists was its ability to kill tumor cells, hence the name). Both IL-1 and TNF-alpha act to increase and perpetuate RA inflammation. Powerful therapies directed at blocking or reducing TNF-alpha are commercially available and widely used.

GETTING DIAGNOSED

Your physician, on hearing that you have joint stiffness, joint pain, fatigue and joint swelling, and finding that the joints are indeed tender and swollen, should suspect RA. However, with more than one hundred different types of arthritis, it can be difficult for a physician to be certain that an arthritis is RA. Because it is so important to get the diagnosis right and to do so early, almost everyone where RA seems possible should see a rheumatologist.

There are features in addition to joint stiffness, pain, swelling, and fatigue that help to correctly diagnose RA: RA usually attacks many joints, it usually attacks the same joints on both sides of the body, and there is an "RA pattern" of *which* joints get attacked.

Typically, once the disease has been present for six weeks, four or more joints are affected. Within months, this number may have escalated to a dozen, to twenty, or even more. Even though only a few of your joints may feel painful early on, an examination by a skilled practitioner will likely reveal mild involvement in others.

When a joint is affected on one side of your body, the same joint tends to be involved on the opposite side. Thus, more often than not, when a knuckle, wrist, knee, or toe on one side of your body is involved, a similar joint on the other is affected. However, the match may not be exact—if your second and third toe on the right are inflamed, it may be the fourth on your left. But this would still be considered as involving the same joint on both sides.

The "RA pattern" means that certain joints are likely to be involved (Fig-

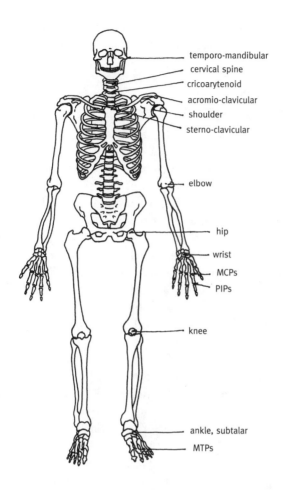

temporo-mandibular
cervical spine
cricoarytenoid
acromio-clavicular
shoulder
sterno-clavicular

elbow

hip

wrist
MCPs
PIPs

knee

ankle, subtalar
MTPs

Fig. 2.2. The pattern of joint involvement in RA. Notable features include: similar joints on both sides of the body are involved (for instance, if the right wrist is inflamed, usually the left wrist also will be affected), and the small joints of the hands are frequently involved, but the last joints of the fingers are spared. With time, more joints become involved.

ure 2.2). These include the *metacarpophalangeal* (MCP), *proximal interphalangeal* (PIP), and wrist joints. The MCP joints are the first row of knuckles as you go down from the wrist, the PIP joints are the second (or middle) row, and the *distal interphalangeal* or DIP joints are the furthest from the wrist. The DIPs are generally not involved in RA. At first diagnosis, the wrists, the MCPs, and the PIPs are each involved on both sides in almost 50 percent of people with RA. Also, the *metatarsophalangeal* or MTP joints (the first row of joints on the toes) are involved in half early on. At the start of the disease, both shoulders or both knees are involved in about one-quarter of cases, and both ankles or both elbows in about one in six. With time, all of these joints are even more likely to be affected. The wrists,

MCPs, and PIPs become affected in at least three-quarters; the MTPs, shoulders, knees, and ankles in half; and the elbows in one-fifth.

RA "CRITERIA"

To help with the diagnosis of RA, the American College of Rheumatology, one of the leading professional societies devoted to arthritis training and research, has developed criteria for RA that are used by physicians world-wide. These were first developed for research purposes so that scientists in Europe, North America, and elsewhere could be certain that what they were calling RA would be the same in studies around the world. While they are not exactly diagnostic criteria, they contain many of the elements of a diagnosis (Table 2.1). If you have been diagnosed as having RA, you probably had at least four of the seven criteria. If any of criteria 1 through 4 are present, they must have been present for at least six weeks to count toward diagnosis. What is immediately apparent is that one can often make the diagnosis of RA without any fancy or expensive lab testing or even X-rays. The first four criteria are all based on the hallmark signs of RA.

The fifth criterion is another clinical feature. *Rheumatoid nodules* are small, usually movable, lumps that are most commonly found on the back of the elbow. They also can be found on the front of the knee, the hands, and less commonly at other pressure points such as the back of the ankle, the head, and the buttocks. Seldom do you see rheumatoid nodules at diagnosis, and less than a third of persons with RA will ever develop these.

The last two criteria are tests. *Rheumatoid factor* is an antibody that is present in minute amounts in almost everyone, and present in larger amounts in people with RA, as well as in people with other inflammatory and chronic infectious diseases. It is called rheumatoid factor because it was first identified in RA. Some call it the "RA test." Its presence does not establish a definitive diagnosis, and for many physicians it confuses as much as it helps. While more than 80 percent of persons with RA will develop a positive test for rheumatoid factor at some point during a lifetime of living with the disease, *only half* will have a positive test early on. In fact, if a physician orders the test without having performed the skilled examination required to assess criteria 1 through 5, the results will likely be misleading. There are more healthy people with rheumatoid factor than there are people who have RA! Thus, a positive rheumatoid factor test is only relevant if you meet several of the first four criteria in Table 2.1.

The other test that is a criterion for RA is X-ray. However, similar X-ray changes to those seen in RA can be seen in other types of arthritis, especially early on, so one cannot rely exclusively on X-ray changes. To add to the difficulty, very few persons with RA will have X-ray changes in the early

**TABLE 2.1. THE 1987 AMERICAN COLLEGE OF RHEUMATOLOGY
CRITERIA FOR RHEUMATOID ARTHRITIS (1)**

Criterion	Definition
1. Morning stiffness	Morning stiffness in and around the joints lasting at least one hour before maximal improvement.
2. Arthritis of three or more joint areas	At least three joint areas have simultaneously had soft tissue swelling or fluid (not just bony overgrowth) observed by a physician. The fourteen possible joint areas are (right and left): proximal interphalangeal (PIP) knuckle joints, metacarpophalangeal (MCP) knuckle joints, wrist, elbow, knee, ankle, and metatarsophalangeal (MTP) toe joints.
3. Arthritis of hand joints	Swelling of the wrist, metacarpophalangeal (MCP) knuckles or proximal interphalangeal (PIP) knuckle joints.
4. Symmetric arthritis	Involvement at the same time of the same joint area on both sides of the body.
5. Rheumatoid nodules	The presence of rheumatoid nodules (lumps) that are actually seen by a physician.
6. Serum rheumatoid factor	Increased amounts of "rheumatoid factor" detected by a test that is rarely positive in healthy individuals (less than 5 percent of healthy persons).
7. X-ray changes	Changes typical of RA on hand and wrist X-rays. These changes must include evidence of damage in an affected joint.

weeks of the disease—in fact, only half will have changes even one year later. Thus, like the rheumatoid factor test, normal X-rays don't rule out the possibility of RA. Although both the rheumatoid factor tests and X-rays are part of the criteria that help establish the diagnosis of RA, they are actually better at predicting how a person will do over the longterm. Persons with RA who have a positive rheumatoid factor or X-rays that show definite RA damage will have more severe disease and will almost certainly need more aggressive treatment.

There is an important lesson here for the person with RA. The news today is filled with reports of medical advances such as new blood tests, new genetic markers, and new machines such as the Magnetic Resonance Imager (MRI). Yet, the diagnosis of RA rests on the physician's skill and, most important, experience. With a skilled physician, your diagnosis will be made promptly. Without a physician or rheumatologist who has the skill to detect multiple tender joints, to detect what may be subtle changes of joint swelling, and to elicit the history of early morning stiffness, no amount of laboratory and X-ray testing will help you get a correct diagnosis. As with most things in life, skill and appropriate experience are not universal qualities of all physicians. Failure to diagnose RA early on can have long-term undesirable consequences, so be vigilant in getting yourself to a rheumatologist—one experienced in RA. See Chapter 3 for helpful information and tips.

RA OUTSIDE OF THE JOINT (EXTRA-ARTICULAR RA)

The principal target for RA is the joint, but RA can attack outside the joint. Over a lifetime with RA, it commonly involves a person's skin, nerves, eyes, and mouth as well. When the disease is more severe, it also can affect the lungs, heart, and blood system, although involvement of these organs is much less common. Fortunately, they respond to aggressive treatment.

Skin

Rheumatoid nodules are one of the official criteria for diagnosing RA. They are movable lumps located in the tissues just under the outer surface of the skin. Occasionally, the nodules are attached to the surface of bone and are not movable. Rarely, they are found in sites located far from a joint, such as the lung. On rare occasions, they can become so large that they interfere with joint function or lead to skin break down, and must be removed surgically. Rheumatoid nodules are usually found in persons who test positive for rheumatoid factor and they are prognostic of more severe disease. They can disappear as the disease is controlled by appropriate treatment.

The cause of the nodules is uncertain, although research suggests that the nodules may form as a result of inflammation of small blood vessels in the tissue just below the skin. When blood vessels become inflamed, this is called a *vasculitis*. If vasculitis involves the skin, a rash can develop that varies from red bumps to actual deep sores (ulcers) in the skin. Very rarely, the vasculitis can become generalized, affecting the bowel, kidney, liver, gut, nerves, and other systems. This generalized vasculitis requires urgent treatment to avoid serious complications or even death.

Eyes and Mouth

The eyes and mouth can become dry due to a decrease in tear and saliva production. This dry eyes (called *keratoconjunctivitis sicca* or *xeroophthalmia*) and dry mouth (*xerostomia*) problem is called Sjögren's syndrome, after Henrik Sjögren, a Danish eye doctor who helped describe it. Sjögren's syndrome can occur in association with other types of arthritis like lupus or can occur alone, but the most common type is in association with RA. Less common symptoms include cough due to dry bronchial tubes (bronchitis sicca), painful sexual intercourse due to vaginal dryness, and trouble swallowing or heartburn due to decreased intestinal secretions. One in six persons with RA will develop at least mild Sjögren's syndrome.

Very rarely, the undersurface of the eye, the sclera, also can become inflammed. This is different from Sjögren's, is very painful, and requires immediate therapy to prevent permanent damage.

Lung

There are multiple types of lung involvement. Scientists don't know why, but lung involvement in RA is twice as common in men as women. Fortunately, lung involvement is usually mild and often causes no symptoms whatsoever. The most common is pleural involvement. The *pleura* is the lining of the lung that separates the lung from the rib cage and muscles. When inflamed, it can cause severe chest pain (pleuritis) and fluid accumulation around the lung (pleurisy). The chest pain is more severe on inhaling. Although sophisticated studies may identify involvement of the lung lining in up to 50 percent of persons with RA, only 20 percent ever develop pain and only 5 percent get a fluid collection. The pleural involvement responds well to treatment.

The next most common lung involvement is a painless thickening of the lung tissue itself (*interstitial fibrosis*). The lung's role is to exchange unneeded carbon dioxide for oxygen and the interstitial tissue is important for this. While subtle changes of interstitial fibrosis are detectable with specialized lung function testing in up to one in three persons with RA, the majority of people never experience symptoms. Over a lifetime of RA, no more than one in seven develop even shortness of breath. Very few need treatment. Because interstitial fibrosis is more common in smokers, smoking is even worse for your overall health if you have RA.

Bronchiolitis, an inflammatory disease of the lung's gas-exchange system, occurs very rarely. It causes severe shortness of breath. Because it is serious, treatment to suppress the inflammation is needed.

Four other types of lung involvement exist. First, rheumatoid nodules occur in the lung in about 1 in 250 persons with RA. The nodules are not dangerous, although sometimes it is necessary to remove them to make certain they are not a cancer. Second, and even more rare, is the combination of RA, rheumatoid nodules in the lung, and coal miner's lung (so-called Caplan's syndrome). Third, the lung can be involved by a generalized vasculitis. Finally, treatment with medication therapies such as methotrexate, gold, D-penicillamine, and cyclophosphamide can cause lung disease in less than 1 percent of people. However, the benefits of methotrexate and gold therapy far outweigh the risk of these medications causing lung disease.

Heart

Similar to the lung, the heart has a lining that protects it from the surrounding tissues. When the lining becomes inflamed, this is called *pericarditis*. With sophisticated testing, up to 30 percent of individuals are found to have developed pericarditis at some point during their life with RA. However, less than 10 percent ever develop symptoms. The most common symptom is chest pain over the front of the chest and breast bone. Pericarditis responds promptly to treatment. In less than 0.5 percent of cases, accumulation of fluid around the heart can compress the heart and necessitate fluid removal and sometimes even surgery.

Blood Supply

We have seen that RA inflammation can spill over from the joint to affect the lung, heart, and other organs. The inflammatory substances and messengers are carried to these organs through the blood supply. Not surprisingly, the blood supply itself can be affected. The inflammatory substances reduce the ability of the bone marrow, the site where blood is made, to produce red blood cells. The resultant low red blood cell count or anemia is usually mild and does not require treatment directed specifically at the anemia.

A much less common but more important result of inflammation in the bloodstream is Felty's syndrome (named after Arthur Felty, a Baltimore physician, who described it). In Felty's syndrome, a number of things happen: the spleen is enlarged; some cells, called *platelets* (cells that help with clotting when one is cut), are often reduced; and the white blood cell count, especially the polymorphonuclear white blood cells, or polys, is reduced. Because the polys play a key role in defending against infection, infections are more common; and there may be deep sores (ulcers) on the legs. Felty's syndrome occurs in less than 1 percent of persons with RA, and usually occurs after ten or more years of severe RA. It responds to treatments such as gold and methotrexate that are directed at RA.

The Nervous System

The most common nerve problem is not a direct attack on the nerve by RA, but compression by mistake. A number of nerves pass through tunnels in the tissues. In normal health, the tunnels protect the nerve from damage. When the tunnels are near joints and tendons, inflammation of the joint or tendon sheath can lead to swelling that compresses the nerve in its tunnel. This can result in a pins-and-needles sensation and weakness. Because the nerve compression in RA arises from inflammation, and because we know that inflammation is worse at rest, these problems often awaken the affected individual from sleep. The most common example is carpal (wrist) tunnel syndrome. In carpal tunnel syndrome, the median nerve is compressed at the wrist. Numbness of the first three digits of the hand on the palm surface result. A similar tarsal (ankle) tunnel syndrome occurs at the ankle w numbness of the sole of the foot. Altogether, there are about half a doz different nerves that can be compressed like those at the wrist and the ankle. Other than the two mentioned, they are rare.

Potentially serious compression of the spinal cord can arise in the neck. The inflammation from RA in the neck can lead to excessive movement between the first and second vertebrae (the main bones of the spine). This can allow the second vertebrae to press on the spinal cord. In less than 0.5 percent of RA, surgery on the neck is needed to prevent irreversible nerve damage.

Finally, in generalized vasculitis, the nerves can be attacked. This results in weakness and a pins-and-needles sensation, usually in the legs. The damage from this can be long-lasting. Fortunately, this is very rare.

The Good News

Because of the large number of organs that can be affected, some scientists prefer the name *rheumatoid disease* to RA, to draw attention to the spread of the disease beyond the joints. Fortunately, with better treatment of RA the frequency of involvement in areas other than the joints appears to be decreasing. For instance, twenty to thirty years ago, most major hospitals kept half a dozen to a dozen beds available just to treat RA, especially the extra-articular problems discussed above. Most hospitals now have no beds reserved for RA. It appears that early aggressive treatment of RA is markedly reducing inflammation in the joints and decreasing the tendency for the disease to spread and cause severe involvement beyond the joints—thus the need for fewer hospitalizations.

HOW RA PROGRESSES

Prompt diagnosis of RA is essential to good long-term control of the disease. The past decade has seen a radical shift in how RA is treated with medications. The old philosophy in administering medication was based on cautious introduction of the very limited number of medication therapies that had been shown to reduce disability from RA. Today, it is recognized that early diagnosis, followed by early aggressive treatment directed at controlling the RA process, is paramount. At any point in the disease, but especially early on, the risk of harm to your body of not treating or ineffectively treating RA far exceeds the risk of side effects from proven beneficial therapies.

Here's why: The inflammation that is the disease results in pain and disability (Figure 2.3). Disability can be physical, which results in difficulty doing things such as dressing, climbing stairs, or working (whether at home or outside the home), but it also can be psychological, which can result in depression or anxiety or both. If the inflammation is controlled, by con-

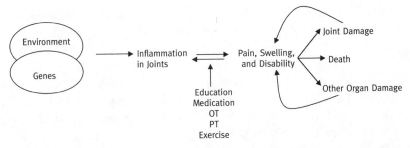

Fig. 2.3. While the exact cause of RA is unknown, the right mix of one's genes and perhaps some exposure such as an infection can trigger the RA inflammation. The inflammation in a joint causes the pain and swelling that results in increasing difficulty using the joint. A variety of interventions including education, medications, physical medicine treatments, occupational therapy, and exercise may reduce the inflammation or counteract the disabling effects of the arthritis. However, if the inflammation goes unchecked, it can cause permanent damage to the joint. Hence, a major aspect of the RA treatment game plan is to diminish and control the inflammation before irreversible damage occurs. Also, continued uncontrolled inflammation can "spill over" to affect other organs such as the eye, lung, lining of the heart, nerves, and so on, and, rarely, it can result in an early death.

trast, pain and disability can be reversed. If the inflammation goes untreated, irreversible damage almost certainly will result (Figure 2.3).

As discussed earlier, damage arises in the joints because the RA inflammation harms the cartilage (the gristle that lines the ends of the bone and allows smooth movement), the bone, and the ligaments and capsule that normally support the joint. Tendons, tendon sheaths, and bursa can all become involved by RA inflammation and contribute to damage. At the present time, short of joint replacement or tendon surgery, joint and tendon damage is permanent. Bursitis also can cause damage, especially in the neck, where it results in the loosening of the vertebrae. Your doctor detects damage by recognizing the joint deformities that commonly result from the uncontrolled inflammation. X-rays also can show permanent damage. This damage is part of a vicious cycle. It causes pain and disability over and above that caused by the inflammation, and both inflammation and damage result is less joint use. This disuse causes muscles to weaken. Weaker muscles provide less support for the joints and further increase the pain and disability. Thus, inflammation, damage, and weak muscles can all cause both pain and disability.

Not only does RA inflammation involve joints, tendons, and bursa, it affects the whole body. In addition to fatigue, inflammation can cause low-grade fever, decreased appetite, and weight loss. If unchecked by treatment, the inflammation can spread to involve other organs, resulting in damage of these organs and adding to disability. Because inflammation starts the process off, it makes sense to detect it early, treat it early, and control or eliminate it early. Fortunately, the past two decades have seen substantial progress and success in our ability to do just that.

Chapter 3

Your Health Care Team

"It's a funny thing about life; if you refuse to accept anything but the best, you very often get it."

—*W. Somerset Maugham*

The PLAN TO WIN involves coming to terms with your RA and believing that you, personally, can affect the outcome of your treatment plan. In the end, it is your fight, and to succeed it's essential to learn everything you can about RA and accept responsibility for the factors within your control.

That doesn't mean, of course, you must face this fight alone. There are all kinds of experienced and dedicated health care professionals ready to help you on your quest for achieving wellness. Ultimately, however, you are in the best position to decide who is on your health care team, and the goals of your treatment plan. After all, only you know what factors are most important to your own health and happiness. Perhaps, for example, you consider pain relief to be your most important goal in the short term, but in the long term, it's important to you to be able to play sports again, or work full-time in a particular occupation. Or maybe your short-term goal is to be able to do daily tasks without having to ask for help, while in the long term, you hope to have a baby. Whatever your individual desires, becoming clear about them will help you decide what help you need and who should provide it.

This chapter is about building the health care "team" that will support you in your efforts to get what you most want from life. Your team roster doesn't necessarily have to involve a long list of players. In fact, you might feel perfectly comfortable with a team of one—trusting entirely in the care and advice provided by your rheumatologist (arthritis specialist). Depending on your situation and the severity of your condition, this may well be your best choice.

In most cases, however, RA creates complications that require the involvement of other specialized health care professionals. These are your team players. Eventually your team will include a personally selected roster of professionals, all focused on the same ultimate goal—your optimal health. Through the course of your disease, your needs and goals will likely change and your team may get larger or smaller, but it should always include a rheumatologist.

BUILDING YOUR HEALTH CARE TEAM

There is no simple method for building a successful health care team. As we have seen in Chapter 2, rheumatoid arthritis is a complex disease and affects everyone differently. Over time, it can change the way it affects even you. The most effective combination of experts on your team depends on your needs, and over time your needs almost certainly will change.

The important thing to remember through all of these changes is that you are the captain of your team. You're the one who provides the focus. It's up to you to set goals, communicate them to the professionals on your team, and provide feedback that will enable others to help you succeed.

The idea of you directing the efforts of a highly trained team of health care professionals might at first seem daunting. They, after all, are the experts. They know the disease and have collectively treated hundreds if not thousands of people with similar symptoms and conditions. You, however, are the expert on *your* condition. No one knows better than you how you feel, what challenges you are facing, what works to relieve your symptoms and what doesn't, and whether at any time your disease is well controlled or not.

By just living with RA and its consequences, you will become intimately familiar with the disease, the effects of various treatments, and the way treatments are used. With time, you can become quite expert at judging your condition and knowing how it's responding to treatment. This first-hand experience, along with your strong personal motivation to succeed, is what makes you the best manager of your treatment plan and the most qualified leader of your health care team.[1]

Accepting responsibility for your health plan can feel overwhelming, especially as you work through the emotions that go with having a chronic disease and all of its impacts. Depending on your personality and the severity of your condition, it can become very tempting to give up, abandoning your role as the manager of your illness and leaving everything to the experts—becoming a passive participant in your own treatment. This may at times feel extremely tempting, but try to be strong and remember, "Never give in." The evidence clearly shows your best chance for successful health outcomes is directly related to your active participation in your treatment plan and to keeping a positive outlook.[2,3]

The skills required of a successful manager are not something you were necessarily born with, but they can be learned. The basic skills are essentially the same whether you're managing situations in the home, in the workplace, or managing the ups and downs of your RA. Ultimately, they amount to:

- planning
- taking responsibility for decisions
- ensuring those decisions are carried out
- monitoring results to maintain steady progress toward a goal

This may sound like one of those things that's easier said than done, but it doesn't have to be difficult. It does, however, require some discipline.

Managing your RA can be made much easier by following these simple guidelines.[4]

Learn as Much as You Can about RA

Your goal is to become the expert on your condition. Start by reading everything you can about RA and using every means possible to become better informed. By reading this book, you are already taking a major step. Visit your local arthritis organization, as well as look up publications, Internet sites, and other resources recommended in Chapter 12. Ask questions of every healthcare professional you visit, and be firm about getting timely and complete answers. The more you know, the greater your sense of control will become.

Pursue Mind-Body Wellness

Rheumatoid arthritis affects more than your physical well-being. In fact, living with RA is bound to have you riding an emotional roller coaster. A regular routine of relaxation and stress-reduction exercises can be helpful for dealing with stress and frustration—which also will help with pain control. So can a network of friends and family with whom you can share your feelings. There is also the option of professional counseling for common issues such as anger, depression, and anxiety (see Chapter 7 for much more on these topics).

Take Responsibility for What You Can Control— and Know What You Can't Control

Taking responsibility involves first acknowledging the things you can't control. Chances are you will have some symptoms and related problems that will not go away in spite of everything you try. These are the things you'll have to work toward accepting as a part of your life with RA. There will be many other aspects of your life still within your control—this is the best place to concentrate your efforts.

Develop a Healthy Lifestyle

Perhaps the best approach to your life with a chronic disease such as RA is to live the life of a healthy person, with all the habits that contribute to a sense of wellness and normality. These include:

- regular exercise
- good nutrition
- plenty of rest
- activities that make you happy
- positive attitude

By adopting the habits of a healthy lifestyle, you can greatly influence the success of your treatment—especially if you can maintain an optimistic outlook. Studies show the power of positive thinking is enormous.

Keep a Health Journal

Another useful strategy for helping you manage your RA is keeping a journal. A health journal offers a great way of keeping track of all the relevant details of your treatment goals, your medications, your response to specific physical, emotional, practical, or mind/body interventions (treatments), and your day-to-day progress. These details provide important information that can be used to more closely tailor treatment to *your* individual needs and aspirations. A journal also can help prepare you for the questions you need to ask during visits to your health professionals. Premade health journals are available through some bookstores, and can even be purchased on-line at www.arthritis.org under the "books" section. A simple spiral bound note pad or blank book will also do the trick nicely. See Chapter 4 for a sample of how to keep track of your medications, dosages, side effects, and progress.

Research has shown that people who keep a written record of their experience with a chronic illness have fewer symptoms, fewer visits to doctors, fewer days off from work, and a more positive outlook than people who don't keep a record.[5] By contrast, there is a concern among some health professionals that journal keeping can become an obsessive behavior, leading to an unhealthy and all-encompassing preoccupation with the disease. The concern is that paying too much attention to symptoms emphasizes illness over wellness. On balance, however, the positives of tracking your experience with RA through some sort of journal far outweigh the negatives.

At the very least, one of the key benefits of a journal is the record it provides to you, the manager of your treatment plan. It also can help you to communicate clearly and consistently with everyone on your health care team, to ensure everyone is working toward the goals that are most important to *you*. A concise record of your current and long-term goals, concerns, medications, symptoms, and treatment experiences ensures everyone on your team is working with the same knowledge and toward the same desired outcomes. It also saves you the time and trouble of having to repeat your story from memory with every new health professional you visit, and gives you a good place to record questions as they arise so you'll have a list ready for your next visit.

A journal also can be useful for identifying things that trigger symptoms or flares. Through regular self-observation and entries in your journal, you can get a clear understanding of your treatment progress and a possible explanation for any fluctuations. The result can be a better understanding of your disease and a heightened sense of control over its progress.

A better understanding of your condition also makes you a better manager of your health care team. With the information collected in your journal, you are well equipped to inform the efforts of everyone on your team.

Lead Your Health Care Team

You are the one managing your treatment, communicating your goals, providing motivation and focus for the team. Research shows that being a passive participant leads to poorer health outcomes—so you do best to take charge, to ensure you get the most from everybody on your team and the best treatment possible for your condition. As well, studies show health care professionals often are more responsive and thorough with patients who are actively involved in their own treatment plans, who follow their health providers' advice, and who communicate regularly and clearly.

YOUR TEAM PLAYERS

So far we've discussed the importance of your taking an active role in your treatment and some of the ways in which this can be done. We've referred to you as the "manager" of your treatment, because it is you who will be guiding the efforts of everyone involved in your care—your treatment team.

In selecting the members of your health care team, you want to engage the best people possible. But where do you start? How can you know who is best for you?

Most people start with their general practitioner, or GP (also referred to as a family doctor), if they already have one. If not, finding a GP is relatively easy. They're listed in the phone book, or you can ask friends or family for recommendations. But selecting a GP is just the starting point for building your treatment team.

In the following pages, we discuss the full range of health care professionals normally associated with the treatment of arthritis. As mentioned earlier, you may begin with a treatment team of one—your rheumatologist.

But over time, it's likely your needs will change and you will be faced with building a larger team of specialists. By becoming familiar with the full range of health care professionals with expertise in RA, along with their different strengths and approaches, you will be in a much better position to make the right choices for your needs and resources.

Medical Practitioners

Doctors play a role in virtually everyone's life. For someone with RA, the importance of that role is huge. And the quality of the relationship you have with your doctors (you are likely to have several doctors on your treatment team at various times) has a direct bearing on the quality of treatment you receive. A survey of arthritis patients' experience with doctors has shown that the more a doctor knows about a person, the greater the effectiveness of their treatment.[6]

The lesson to draw from this is that it is imperative that you feel satisfied with your relationship with your doctor. It should be a relationship based on trust, and backed by a feeling of confidence in his/her abilities. If you don't feel this way about your doctor, it's probably time to find a new one.

The decision to find a new doctor is always yours to make. There is no reason to stay with a doctor if you feel dissatisfied or uncomfortable in that relationship. We suggest that you treat changing your doctor in the same way you might change your lawyer or accountant. Although there are undeniable advantages to maintaining a long-term professional relationship, those benefits amount to little if, at a personal level, you are unhappy with the relationship or aren't getting the outcomes you desire.

Having said that, most people with arthritis report a very high level of satisfaction with their doctors.[7] If there is any concern, it is with the limited time they are able to spend with their doctors. However, the same study has shown most people accept this as a normal consequence of a doctor's busy schedule and, in spite of it, are still quite satisfied with the quality of treatment they receive.

GENERAL PRACTITIONER (GP)

After the common cold and other upper respiratory tract infections, musculoskeletal conditions such as arthritis are the most common cause for people to consult a health professional, so every general practitioner (GP) has almost certainly seen patients with RA coming into their office.[8] Unfortunately, however, during their medical schooling, GPs receive little or no training in the diagnosis and treatment of arthritis—and there are over one hundred types, of which RA is only one. One study has reported only 3 percent of a doctor's preclinical training is given to the entire subject of musculoskeletal diseases.[9]

Although your GP should be able to answer basic questions about arthritis and make some recommendations on treatment, few are expert in inflammatory arthritis. In the case of RA, this caution applies even more strongly. Rheumatoid arthritis is notoriously difficult to diagnose and can progress rapidly if not treated promptly with appropriate medications. Most GPs are aware of this and should refer you to a rheumatologist if they suspect you have an arthritis such as RA. If no referral is suggested, you should insist on it.

As you start to assemble your treatment team of experts, your dependence on your GP may decline. However, he or she still has an important role to play as a primary care physician receiving up-to-date reports on all the care you receive for your arthritis, perhaps helping to administer medications or monitor test results, and assisting with many of the non-RA related reasons you may need to see a doctor from time to time.

In a health care world populated by innumerable specialists, GPs are the generalists. The wide range of their experience and training means they can relate well to the other members of your health care team. This allows them to play an important coordinating role on your behalf. It also means, where required, they can refer you to health care specialists you may not be aware of.

Communication among the members of your team is also important. To keep your treatment focused and moving in the right direction, everyone on your team must work together toward the same goals. This requires communication, which is something your GP can help you to achieve.

One final point: Osteopaths are, by general training, similar to GPs in their medical expertise. Thus, osteopaths can provide diagnoses, prescribe drugs, and perform surgery, but are not well equipped through their training to diagnose and treat RA.

INTERNIST

Internists are the least specialized of the medical specialists. Unlike GPs, they do not treat children, assist women through childbirth, perform minor surgery or set fractures. Their focus is all internal medicine (adult diseases), so arthritis is just one of many conditions they are trained to diagnose and treat. Increasingly in the United States, internists play an oversight role, taking on the activities of a GP, and coordinating the care for persons with chronic disease. In situations where a rheumatologist is unavailable, internists can provide general care and treatment for RA, but their limited arthritis training means they are far less qualified to successfully diagnose and treat the disease, unless they have taken extra training.

RHEUMATOLOGIST

Rheumatologists are specialists in the diagnosis and treatment of arthritis. While a GP will have one or two years' training after medical school, a rheumatologist will have completed three years' training in internal medicine, and then at least two or three years' training solely focused on arthritis. A rheumatologist will have spent more time learning how to read X-rays of joints than a radiologist. They will have spent much more time learning about arthritis medications than a pharmacist. A rheumatologist who is up-to-date on RA will know, from attendance at conferences and congresses, about new treatments months before they are published in medical journals and years before they appear in medical textbooks. In that RA is one of the most severe and disabling of the more than one hundred types of arthritis, this extensive training is likely to be essential in getting the best advice in a timely manner.

Given a rheumatologist's expertise with arthritis, it comes as no surprise that in a clinical survey of arthritis patients, rheumatologists were found to provide more relief from the symptoms of arthritis than any other health care professional.[10] People with RA under the care of rheumatologists also experience better long-term health outcomes through their treatment. However, we do suggest that, if at all possible, you see a rheumatologist who has a major interest and experience in RA (as opposed to one of many other forms of arthritis, such as lupus, fibromyalgia, or osteoarthritis). Ideally, your rheumatologist will be treating one hundred or more people with RA.

During the early period after diagnosis, your rheumatologist will probably want to see you once or twice a month. Among other things, he or she will use these visits to assess progress in severity or improvement of your RA, and to monitor results (including negative side effects) from your medication.

ORTHOPEDIC SURGEON

Many people with RA may never require surgery. If you should ever need surgery for removal of inflamed tissue around joints or tendons, replacement of a damaged joint, or surgery on a joint because of pain, poor quality of life, or risk of serious damage or deformity, you are likely to see an orthopedic surgeon. For hand surgery, it may be a plastic surgeon, and for neck disease, it may be a neurosurgeon. Your rheumatologist should be able to advise you on the qualifications and experience of different surgeons. Surgery also can be used to relieve pressure on nerves in the neck or wrists.

Orthopedic surgeons are doctors specially trained to perform surgical treatment on joints, bones, tendons, and ligaments—in fact, everything concerned with the movement of your body. Like rheumatologists, orthopaedic surgeons have at least six or seven years of specialized training after medical school. Of course, orthopedic surgeons deal with all kinds of conditions (some do only trauma surgery or spinal surgery), so in choosing your surgeon, make sure he or she is specialized in treating people with arthritis.

Where required, surgery can be extremely effective in providing relief from pain and restoring mobility to affected joints. While nonsurgical treatments are generally favored over surgery, don't think of it as a last resort. Even at an early stage of your treatment plan, if inflammation in a joint is causing pressure on a nerve or the joint is damaged, surgery can sometimes be the most effective way of reducing pain and restoring joint mobility.

For more information on surgery, see Chapter 10.

NURSE

Nurses often have much to offer as a part of your health care team. Many of the medications prescribed for RA are powerful ones with possible side effects. An arthritis nurse can take an active role in medication monitoring, using blood and urine tests to make sure you get the full benefit of your therapy with a minimum of side effects. Nurses also are often called on to administer medication, especially medicine that requires injection. Or, if you prefer self-injection, your nurse is probably the best person to show you how.

Allied Health Practitioners

OCCUPATIONAL THERAPIST (OT)

Don't be misled by the term "occupational." Occupational therapists, or OTs, are not just overly concerned with your paid working life. Of all the members of your health care team, your OT probably has the most practical role of all. It's their job to show you how to handle the demands of everyday life and get things done with a minimum of pain, stress, and fatigue.

Self-care, personal hygiene, leisure, recreation, work—the activities of normal life all require a level of physical adeptness most people take for granted. But with RA, nothing can be taken for granted. Even the simplest tasks, such as buttoning a shirt, opening a jar, or tying a shoe, can be excruciatingly difficult. With the help of your OT, however, you can find practical solutions for virtually any problem, as well as the means for achieving a level of independence that might otherwise be impossible.

On your first visit to an OT, you can expect a lot of questions. In assessing your situation, your OT will want to know what kinds of activities are painful or difficult and how often you perform them. They also may want to know about your medication, past surgeries, and any other health conditions that may be relevant (e.g, diabetes, heart or lung disease, etc.).

Your OT will want to identify every area affected by your RA and determine your comfortable range of motion. An OT may ask about home and work environments, about the help available to you from family and friends, and about your financial situation. All of these considerations are required for determining the best solutions for your individual needs.

Almost every intervention an OT performs is focused on two primary concerns: joint protection and energy conservation. Guided by these principles, your OT will likely spend time teaching you practical strategies. Looking at your daily routine, for example, your OT will assist you to prioritize and schedule activities for when your energy levels are highest. He or she will also provide tips on how and when to effectively work rest breaks into your routine.

Joint protection might involve recommendations for adaptive equipment or specific tools designed to make an activity easier to perform. Depending on your condition, splinting may be required to protect and rest a joint with RA, usually a wrist or a hand. (See Chapter 9, for more information about splinting.)

At some point, your OT may suggest a home or work visit—and you may do well to take them up on this offer. A home or work assessment may be the single most helpful thing an OT can provide. An OT can suggest all kinds of aids and devices to increase your independence and make your life easier—everything from specially designed can or bottle openers to long-handled shoehorns that eliminate the need to bend or stoop. In the workplace, an OT can provide suggestions for adapting your environment to make it more friendly for you.

Your OT is a trained and highly specialized problem solver. For any task made difficult by RA, look to your OT for solutions. If the troublesome task requires an implement not commercially available, it can be built. No problem is too small.

PHYSIOTHERAPIST (PT)

Depending on the severity of your disease, your physiotherapist (also referred to as physical therapist, or PT) is someone with whom you could wind up spending a lot of time. When your disease is most active, a typical treatment regime might include three, forty-five-minute visits a week. Under these circumstances, chances are you'll get to know your PT pretty well, and vice versa.

Physical therapy has a long history of association with arthritis. Indeed, many of the principal tools of the physiotherapist for treating arthritis—movement, massage, heat, cold, electricity, and water—are the same today as in centuries past.

A first visit to a PT should involve a comprehensive assessment. The physiotherapist will want to know everything related to your experience with RA, as well as any other medical history.

The next step is a physical examination. Your PT will assess the range of motion for all joints of your body, measure the muscle strength of your major joints and your affected joints, and examine affected joints for swelling, stability, and any other factors.

Based on your medical history and physical exam, your PT will then propose a plan for your physiotherapy. This is a collaborative process—it requires your input and your consent, and it will only succeed if you understand and agree to it. As part of the plan, goals will be set and treatment will continue until those goals are met or your progress reaches a plateau.

Given the amount of time you spend with your PT, you can expect to hear a great deal about the importance of maintaining a balance between rest and activity. They'll also let you know about the principles behind resting and the difference between general rest, and specific rest for a particular joint.

PTs can also help correct misguided notions. For example, exercising a knee that is hot and swollen by going up and down stairs will not, as some people might think, help it recover. In fact, such exercise can be the very worst thing for a hot swollen joint.

For pain associated with RA, PTs rely on two main treatments: cold and electricity. By reducing heat and inflammation, ice packs can provide short-term pain relief, allowing a person to perform exercises that would otherwise be impossible. Electrical treatment is used to stimulate certain nerves, affecting their ability to transmit the sensation of pain. Electrical stimulation is also thought to trigger the release of endorphins, which are hormones produced by the body that act as natural painkillers.

The most important area of physical therapy is exercise, which is done for three reasons:

- to maintain or improve range of motion
- to maintain or improve muscle strength
- to improve a person's overall physical condition

Range-of-motion exercises

These are very light exercises with an emphasis on taking the joints through the fullest extent of motion possible. This kind of exercise should be done daily by people with RA to avoid losing mobility in their affected joints.

Strength exercises

These exercises are done to preserve or increase muscle strength and bulk and require the use of resistance. Isometric exercises strengthen muscles by tensing them without putting stress on or moving the joint.

General conditioning exercises

Twenty years ago, the idea of someone with RA exercising to maintain their general fitness was almost unknown. Today, the benefits of fitness for people with RA are proven through research.

For more depth on the above topics, please see Chapter 5.

CHOOSING AN OCCUPATIONAL THERAPIST OR PHYSICAL THERAPIST

In choosing an OT or PT, look for someone who has experience with RA, and preferably some specialized training. In general practice, some OTs and PTs may not see a person with RA more than once a year. Be sure to ask.

It's also important to find an OT or PT you feel comfortable with and can relate well to on a personal level. Given the amount of time you'll be spending with this person, it's important to choose someone you like. That way, as you open up to your physiotherapist, sharing your hopes, fears, and concerns, you can get the full value of their experience.

Your local arthritis organization (Arthritis Foundation in Australia and the United States; The Arthritis Society in Canada; Arthritis Care in United Kingdom; and the Arthritis Foundation of New Zealand (Inc.)), will most likely be able to provide references to OTs and PTs experienced in treating RA. For contact information, please see "Associations for People with Arthritis" in Chapter 12.

PHYSIATRIST

Physiatry is probably the least well known area of medicine. But for people with severe arthritis needing lots of rehabilitation, the physiatrist can make a big difference.

A physiatrist (pronounced *fizz-EYE-a-trist*) is a medical doctor, a specialist in physical medicine, and an authority on exercise and rehabilitation. As with other members of a potential team, some physiatrists may have less experience with RA. It is best to find a physiatrist experienced in the long-term care of people with RA.

Their approach is to use physical treatments such as water, ice, heat, and electrical stimulation. They often play a supervisory role on the rehabilitation team, directing the activities of OTs and PTs.

PHARMACIST

Medications are still the most effective treatment for RA. While pharmacists are experts at dispensing medications, relatively few people give much thought to other types of help a pharmacist can provide as a member of their health care team.

If you have problems or side effects with your medication and can't see your rheumatologist or general practitioner right away, try speaking with your pharmacist. He or she may be able to answer some of your medication-related questions. A good pharmacist, for example, will be able to tell whether your side effects are serious or not. For advice about changing medications or dosages, however, see your rheumatologist.

In choosing a pharmacist, look for the same qualities you'd want from your medical practitioners. You will probably be having a long-term association with this person, so it's important to choose someone you trust and can talk to easily. Staying with the same pharmacist is a good idea, because it means they'll be able to keep a record of your prescriptions and can look out for possible drug interactions. They also can help by advising you on less costly generic versions of the medications you're taking.

Some pharmacists are more familiar with the kinds of medication prescribed for RA than others. If you have trouble finding a pharmacist knowledgeable about medication therapies for RA, try asking your rheumatologist. They're bound to know of pharmacies catering to the prescription needs of their patients with RA.

PODIATRIST

Over time, almost all people with RA develop problems with their feet, causing pain that makes walking difficult.

Podiatrists provide treatment for problems of the feet. The solutions they offer range from orthotics and prescription-molded shoes for simple problems to surgery for correcting deformities, bunions, misaligned bones, crooked toes, or pinched nerves.

An experienced podiatrist is also able to differentiate foot problems related to RA from other types that may appear to be similar. This distinction is important, as arthritis-related foot problems may require different treatment.

OPHTHALMOLOGIST

An ophthalmologist is a physician with special training in the medical and surgical aspects of eye disorders. An ophthalmologist may be needed to help with dry eyes, which can be a problem for some people with RA. Examinations by ophthalmologists are essential to preventing side effects from antimalarial medications used to treat RA. They may be needed to treat cataracts that can occur due to cortisone and related medications.

NUTRITIONIST OR REGISTERED DIETICIAN

Like many people with RA, you may have concerns about your diet and its effect on your condition. You may be concerned, for example, that your food is interacting with your medication, or you may be having weight problems due to your medication and a reduced level of physical activity. As well, you may be wondering if any foods are known to worsen or improve RA symptoms.

Be careful about whom you go to for answers to these concerns. Although many people can claim to be knowledgeable about diet and nutrition, it's best to consult a professional. A qualified nutritionist or registered dietitian is a trained and highly skilled professional and can provide helpful and reliable advice on everything to do with food and nutrition. For essential information on diet and RA, see Chapter 6.

CLINICAL PSYCHOLOGISTS AND SOCIAL WORKERS

Rheumatoid arthritis may force many changes in your life. Most of those changes will be physical, but RA also can affect you psychologically and socially. The role of a psychologist or social worker is to help you deal with those changes to ensure you experience a healthy emotional and psychological adjustment to your life with RA.

People deal with distress in different ways. Some are able to work through their feelings and practical issues on their own or with the help of close family and friends. Others may prefer having the professional support that a trained psychologist or social worker can offer.

People newly diagnosed with RA typically have five basic issues they must face.[11] The first is coping with a sense of loss. Obviously there's a physical loss, but there also may be loss of income, loss of social and recreational opportunities, and lost dreams for the future—or fear of such losses.

Emotional reactions to that sense of loss can include anger, depression, and fear.

Insufficient social support can also be an issue for some people. Perhaps you feel you have nobody to talk to. Or you may not feel comfortable talking with your family or friends at the level of intimacy and openness required for dealing with personal problems. A psychologist or social worker can offer the practiced ear and helpful advice you may find difficult requesting or obtaining from family and friends.

Finally, some people with RA develop low self-esteem. As they encounter more and more activities made difficult by their RA, they may start to feel incompetent and lose their sense of confidence and control.

Psychologists and social workers are trained to help you recognize and work through these feelings, and assist you to build on your strengths. Their goal is to help you regain confidence in your ability to manage your life and your RA.

Social workers can help you gain access to appropriate programs and supports available through government agencies and other organizations. They can help you work through financial problems, find suitable housing, or get job retraining should you require it.

Psychologists provide professional counseling for emotional and personal areas of your life. A psychologist can, for example, teach you mind-body techniques for relaxation and pain management. Using techniques such as cognitive behavioral therapy, self-hypnosis, imagery, biofeedback, and relaxation, a psychologist can help you use your mind to break the cycle of stress, sleep disturbance and pain. Psychologists also can help you with sexual, relationship, and emotional issues (such as anger, depression and anxiety), related to your RA.

For an in-depth exploration of emotions and RA, please see Chapter 7.

Complementary Health Practitioners

The number of unproven and unusual treatments that people with RA have tried over the years shows the depth of their frustration in finding relief through more conventional treatments. The desire for a miracle cure has led to all kinds of questionable remedies. People have tried everything from bee venom and honey to copper bracelets and WD-40 lubricating oil.

In spite of the endless array of bizarre and unproven approaches, there is an area of treatment for arthritis outside the field of orthodox medicine that has achieved widespread acceptance. These nonmedical health practitioners provide treatment that many people with RA have found effective, and that even some parts of the medical community have come to acknowledge as legitimate.

We consider these approaches to be "complementary" health practices, because they offer treatment that can complement (but not replace) the treatment you receive from your rheumatologist and team of health professionals.

MASSAGE THERAPIST

Massage is probably the simplest approach to the physical treatment of RA and, for some people, has been shown to reliably offer pain relief.[12] If done improperly, however, it can have negative consequences and potentially cause physical damage. If you wish to try massage, your best approach is to seek a licensed massage therapist with experience in treating many people with RA.

ACUPUNCTURIST

Acupuncture has been practiced as a healing art for thousands of years in China. Although researchers are still undecided about exactly *how* acupuncture works, there is no dispute that it does work—though not for all people. In one clinical survey of people with arthritis, acupuncture was found to provide long-term pain relief for just over half the people surveyed.[13]

The same study revealed that not all acupuncturists are equally skilled in their mastery of this ancient practice.

Make sure your acupuncturist is both licensed and experienced in the technique. A medical doctor who dabbles in acupuncture is much less likely to provide the relief you seek than a nonmedical practitioner fully trained in the theory and use of acupuncture. And, of course, be sure your acupuncturist works only with new needles taken from sterile packages.

If you do decide to try acupuncture for your RA, *don't abandon your medications*. For actively inflamed joints, acupuncture is no substitute for medication, which provides much more reliable results. Plus, suspending or delaying medication therapy has been shown to dramatically increase the risk of permanent joint damage. While acupuncture can help some with pain arising from damaged joints, it cannot reverse the underlying cause of your illness or cure your RA.

Acupuncture is considered a safe treatment, with no appreciable side effects. It can, however, be expensive. If your insurance plan doesn't cover the cost, you will be paying between $25 and $70 a treatment, and you may need ten to twenty visits before you notice any improvement.

Alternative Remedies

Many people with RA take alternative remedies such as glucosamine, chondroitin, and vitamins, and they ask about the potential effectiveness of ginger, MSM, green tea, fish oil, selemium, and echinacea (which is, actually, dangerous for people with RA). If you are interested in learning more about these or other remedies, we recommend that you consult *The Arthritis Foundation's Guide to Alternative Therapies* (The Arthritis Foundation, 1999). In the interim, however, we emphatically recommend against using any complementary or alternative treatments as a replacement for your primary medical treatment. (See Chapter 6 for more on this topic.)

Getting the Most from Your Relationships With Health Professionals

As a person with a chronic illness you will, of course, be spending a lot of time with health professionals: GPs, rheumatologists, physiotherapists, and the like. And as the manager of your treatment, you are the one to decide which professionals you want on your team. It's possible to simplify the decision process for selecting a health professional down to two main considerations: professional suitability and personal fit.

Professional Suitability

By professional suitability, we mean the *kind* of health professional required, that is, their area of specialization (for example, RA management, surgery, clinical psychology) and their level of competence. Earlier in this chapter, we reviewed the types of doctors most usually consulted for the treatment of RA. Foremost among such doctors, of course, are rheumatologists. But there are other health professionals you also may want to involve, and in every case you should be careful in appraising their experience and professional suitability for your situation.

Many people are intimidated by health professionals, however, and it can be difficult to ask a professional for his or her qualifications. But it's essential you know the track record and skills of anyone you are going to hire to be on your team. Whether the bill will be paid by your insurance, taxes, or out of pocket, *you are paying*, and you deserve and need to know what you are getting. After all, it's your *health* that's at stake. Plus, you'll be showing the practitioner that you're serious about your care and you have high expectations of his or her performance.

Following are some of the questions you might ask in assessing a health professional's qualifications before selecting him or her to join your health care team.

- What is your experience in treating people with RA?
- How many RA patients are you actively treating? (For rheumatologists, physiotherapists and so on, the answer should be more than one hundred on a regular basis.)
- How long have you been in practice?
- How do you stay up-to-date on new RA treatments?
- Are you part of a specialized clinic or group practice where you have the benefit of interaction with colleagues?

Personal Fit

Personal fit is the other important consideration. Given the amount of time and the degree of trust you will be investing in your relationship with your health professionals, it's imperative you feel good about those relationships. Your team members have to be people who feel right for you. Of course, the "right feeling" means different things to different people. Some people may prefer brisk efficiency from their health professionals, while others may need more warmth and personability. There is no "one size fits all." We all have different personalities with different needs. You are the only one who can decide on the professionals who best fit with your personal needs.

A HEALING RELATIONSHIP

There is one thing, however, that everyone should demand continually from their health professionals: a "healing relationship."[14] This means having them relate to you as a person, before relating to your disease. It's very easy for health professionals—doctors, in particular—to neglect this important aspect of the relationship, trained as they are in the technology of medicine and the clinical approach, and pressured by limitations of time.

You can help set the right tone by making sure your health professional knows more about you than just your symptoms and the information on your chart. A healing relationship requires that your health professional is aware of everything that may be affecting your health, including things such as your aspirations and anxieties and your personal strengths and weaknesses.

A word of caution is perhaps required here. Finding a health professional who matches your needs for both professional qualification and personal fit is not an automatic guarantee of top-notch medical treatment. If you've put a premium on choosing a health professional for his or her personal style, you may have overlooked their shortcomings on experience or technical competence. Conversely, a prestigious degree and first-rate credentials might ensure great technical competence but don't necessarily make a great caregiver. In a very general sense, the best health professional is one who combines up-to-date knowledge with depth of experience and a desire to treat "the whole you." In such cases, the probable outcome is a health professional with good judgment. And that's the best qualification of all.[15]

Visiting Your Health Professional

Most health professionals are busy individuals. The demands of a professional practice means they must be fairly efficient in their approach to patients. Health professionals will do their best to ensure they understand your situation and your needs, but their knowledge is essentially limited to what you share. That means it's up to you to make sure you get everything you need from your visit. Most health professionals appreciate patients who are forthright about their problems and show an interest in learning more about their condition. Although it may require some extra time and effort for your health professional to address all your concerns initially, over the longer term it will almost certainly save time and perhaps even reduce the number of visits you require.

Before the Visit

Begin by being prepared. Following is a list of helpful tips:[16,17]

- if you're starting with a new medical doctor (such as a rheumatologist or orthopaedic surgeon), arrange to have copies of your medical records sent to their office before your visit
- bring any recent X-rays
- think carefully about what you want the health professional to know about you and your reasons for seeking treatment—Be specific, for instance, "My goal is to be able to work five half-days a week as a bus driver"

- write down all your questions and take them with you for the visit
- highlight your most important questions, as you may not have time in one visit to get answers for all of them
- if this is a repeat visit, prepare a summary of what has happened since your last visit; make a copy to leave with your health professional
- make sure you know the names and dosages of all the medications you're taking
- if you're visiting your rheumatologist, note any prescription refills you might need
- be prepared to discuss any side effects of your current treatment or medication

In the Health Professional's Office

Remember your role as the manager of your treatment plan. You are not there to simply hear and obey. Your active participation and direction is important to achieving the results you're after.

One way you can demonstrate your role as an active partner and manager of your health care team is to request access to your file. This is perfectly within your rights and allows you the comfort of knowing everything your health professional knows about you and your condition.

When visiting your health professional, if it makes you more comfortable, or you think you might not remember everything said, consider bringing a friend or family member. That way, you can discuss the appointment afterward to make sure you understood everything your health professional said. You might even consider using a tape recorder during the appointment to ensure nothing is forgotten. Particularly when pain, fatigue, depression or anxiety are present, it can be difficult to take in a lot of complex information or advice at once.

Another useful idea is repeating back to your health professional everything told to you, including diagnosis, prognosis, treatment, and recommendations. This can help you understand and remember everything after you leave the office.

Make sure your health professional knows about your experiences with other members of your health care team. The more information your health professional has about your condition and the full range of your treatment experience, the better. Of course, the same rule applies for all the members of your team. The more they know about each other and your experience, the better informed their recommendations will be.

Many people feel unable to ask their most important questions or to raise their most pressing concerns at the start of an appointment. You may, for example, feel more comfortable starting with simple questions before launching into more personal topics. This, however, could lead your health professional to misinterpret the urgency or priority of your concerns. Another approach is to mention to your health professional that you have a list of important questions, and to ask whether it's best to deal with those questions before or after the examination or treatment.

If your doctor recommends tests, be sure to ask what the tests are for and how much they cost. This is one sure way to let your doctor know you are an active partner in the process. If the rationale for the test seems weak or the results can't be directly related to your treatment, don't be afraid to question whether it's really necessary. (Chapters 2 and 4 provide information about RA tests.)

Similarly, make sure you explore all treatment options with your health professional. And remember, doing nothing is always an option. Before accepting any treatment, you should know everything possible about it—all its pros and cons and the reasons why your health professional is recommending it for your disease. It's possible you might disagree with a treatment recommendation based on what you know about yourself and your RA. If that's the case, a mutually acceptable alternative can usually be found.

Ultimately, it's up to you to decide on your course of treatment. Your team members will provide recommendations, but unless you accept them as offering what's best for you, you're unlikely to follow through. The result could very well compromise the success of your treatment.

There will always be complementary and alternative therapies. For as long as people have suffered the aching pains of RA, there have been "remedies"—some more orthodox than others. It is always up to you whether you choose to pursue one of these treatments. But it is also important that you let your doctor or rheumatologist know about any other treatment you engage in. For one thing, there could be dangerous interactions with medications you are taking. It's also important that you continue following his or her treatment advice as well. (There is more on this in Chapter 4.)

This raises the issue of "compliance." Superficially, it means doing exactly what your health professional tells you. And were you to do that without questioning, you would hardly be the manager of your treatment plan. What's more, without understanding the reasons behind your health professional's advice, it's much less likely you would actually follow that advice very closely.

In one study of people with arthritis, it was found that although patients were generally compliant, almost half reported only taking their medication when they were experiencing pain or inflammation. Along similar lines, another study showed that more than half the participants did not follow their doctor's prescribed therapy closely enough for it to be effective.[18,19]

The key here is your full understanding of the advice given by your rheumatologist. This is essential. For example, if you are fully aware of all the benefits of your medication, which may include disease suppression along with pain relief, you are far more likely to take the medication as prescribed. As well, you will better understand the possible consequences of nonadherence, such as the potential for permanent joint damage and deformity.

Your willingness to comply with professional advice is also more likely if you are asked to provide input. This is something you should expect from your health professional. For example, in talking about any medication, your doctor should provide a full explanation of everything it entails: the reasons for the medication, the importance of dosage and frequency, and any possible side effects. The same is true of exercises recommended by your physiotherapist, or therapies prescribed by other members of your team. If the recommended therapy or possible side effects make you uncomfortable, ask about other treatment options. By taking a role in deciding which therapies are right for you, you can ensure that your treatment plan truly is *your* plan.

Chapter 4

MEDICATIONS

"Most of the fundamental ideas of science are essentially simple, and may,
as a rule, be expressed in a language comprehensible to everyone."

—Albert Einstein

Today, there is unanimity amongst rheumatologists worldwide that for persons with even mild RA, medication therapy forms an essential part of their treatment plan. However, for you—the person with RA—making the decision to include medication therapy can be difficult.

Arming yourself with information on available medications will help you to make informed decisions about which one (or which combination) you should include in your treatment plan. Knowing what medications are commonly used; how they work; what their potential benefits and possible side effects are; how they are taken; and what they cost—all are factors to consider before making your decision.

Although no medication available today "cures" RA, there are a number that have been proven safe and effective. For the vast majority of people with RA, these therapies help restore their ability to care for themselves and their family, the ability to resume or continue to work, and the ability to enjoy physical activity again. In other words, the ability to maintain or regain quality of life.

But remember, just like snowflakes, no two people with RA are identical—they will have different symptoms, prognoses, and treatment plans. The plan you create with your health care team should be designed to meet your specific needs.

EARLY, AGGRESSIVE MEDICATION THERAPY

Starting early, aggressive medication therapy is the most important thing you can do to achieve long-term optimal health with RA. Of all the components in your treatment plan, only medication therapy has been scientifically proved effective at slowing or halting RA. But deciding to include early, aggressive medication therapy as part of your treatment plan may not be easy, especially if you are newly or recently diagnosed.

For most individuals, facing the diagnosis of RA and determining what it will mean to their life is challenge enough in the early going. If this rings true for you, we encourage you to read this section carefully. Understanding the rationale behind early, aggressive medication therapy will help you gain insights into your disease and your rheumatologist's recommendations, and can help you make informed decisions at a time when the world seems upside down.

RESEARCH TELLS THE STORY

Prior to the mid-1980s, the customary medication therapy was a highly conservative one: individuals with RA were treated with aspirin (salicylates) or a *nonsteroidal anti-inflammatory drug* (NSAID) for up to a year—or more—before stronger *disease-modifying anti-rheumatic drugs* (DMARD) were initiated. When DMARD therapy was finally started, the person remained on the therapy even if the benefits were minimal.

This "go slow" practice was, in large part, because few DMARDs existed before 1980. Rheumatologists hesitated to move a person with a chronic, lifelong disease down the medication therapy list too quickly. The conservative approach continued up to the late 1980s, even though new DMARDs became available. But evidence began to mount that "going slow" produced disastrous results for the person with RA.

A number of research studies in the late 1980s looked at conservatively treated individuals' health over a number of years. One, a landmark 1987 study, tracked the same 112 individuals from the time of diagnosis over a twenty-year period. It reported sobering results: although the 112 were mainly young women, thirty-seven, or a staggering 33 percent, were dead within twenty years. (None of the deaths could be directly attributed to DMARD therapy.) Of the survivors at the end of twenty years, 38 percent had severe incapacity; another 26 percent were housebound or bedridden.[1]

Other studies following severe RA showed that conservative treatment resulted in premature death at a rate equal to that of severe heart disease or Hodgkin's lymphoma (lymphatic cancer).[2] Additional research showed inflammation from RA caused significant permanent joint damage and loss of function within the first two years after the disease started.[3]

Pieced together, mounting evidence began to tell an alarming story: The long-term results of conservative medication therapy were permanent disability or premature death for the vast majority with RA. Clearly, change to the medication approach was needed fast. Yet, change was slow to come.

Why? One reason rheumatologists delayed or avoided initiating DMARD therapy was because of concern over side effects. In the absence of research comparing the relative *toxicity* (potential for side effects) of NSAIDs and DMARDs, it was widely believed that NSAIDs were the safer of the two. It is now recognized that the toxicity of the two are similar, even though DMARDs can lead to disease control and NSAIDs cannot. In fact, some DMARDs (e.g., hydroxychloroquine) are actually safer than NSAIDs.

A NEW APPROACH:
START EARLY, BE AGGRESSIVE, GET BETTER

By 1990, a new medication therapy plan emerged. Researchers and rheumatologists recognized that swollen joints were a key marker for future disability (difficulty with most activities of daily living, like walking and working) and eventual permanent joint damage. So, controlling inflammation and resultant swelling as early and completely as possible became the number one goal. At the heart of the new approach were these concepts:

1. Medication therapy with DMARDs should begin as early as possible after RA starts.
2. DMARD therapy should be maintained.
3. If necessary, combinations of DMARDs should be used when one DMARD alone is unable to control disease symptoms.

Over a decade later, the question is: Does the new approach work? Research resoundingly says, Yes.

A half-dozen studies looking at the short-term benefits of early DMARD therapy reported that DMARD treatment in individuals within months of the start of RA showed significant improvement from symptoms compared to those on placebo ("dummy" or sugar pills). In addition, two studies, one from Europe[4] and one from Canada,[5] looked at the long-term benefits of early DMARD therapy. One study reported that even a delay of six to nine months in starting DMARD therapy led to uncontrolled joint swelling, joint damage, and disability; the other study reported similar results after nine months.

Finally, a long-term study from centers in the United States and Canada showed that individuals who maintained the DMARD therapy faired significantly better than those treated with the older conservative approach. In fact, more consistent DMARD use lessened long-term disability by 30-percent.[6] In real life, a 30-percent improvement meant that an individual confined to bed would be out of bed and walking with a cane, or someone using a cane would be living a near "normal" life. These are huge advances.

COMBINATION MEDICATION THERAPY

The final proposal to control RA disease, to control it early and completely, was to use combinations of DMARDs along with NSAIDs. The combination medication therapy centers on the use of two or more DMARDs at the same time without increasing toxicity.

For years, combination medication therapy has proved key in controlling other chronic conditions such as heart disease, high blood pressure, asthma, HIV/AIDS, as well as slowing or curing cancer. In these conditions, not all combinations work. Indeed, recent studies in RA show that some DMARD combinations do not provide added benefit, or do so at the cost of increased toxicity. Examples of unsuccessful combinations are the combinations of antimalarial medications with D-penicillamine, or methotrexate with azathioprine. However, other DMARD combinations do provide the person with RA benefit, with little or no increase in side effects. The best examples of these would be intramuscular gold with hydroxychloroquine; methotrexate with sulphasalazine and hydroxychloroquine; cyclosporine-A plus methotrexate; etanercept and methotrexate; infliximab with methotrexate, and leflunomide with methotrexate.

Studies exploring other combinations will determine if they provide greater benefit in combination or as a single therapy, thus potentially expanding the number of medication treatment options for the person with RA. The list of successful combinations is sure to grow.

PATIENCE IS A VIRTUE

This age-old adage could not be truer. It may take time to find the right therapy, or combination of therapies, that works best against your RA. Try not to be discouraged if the first couple of therapies your rheumatologist recommends do not produce the desired results. RA symptoms and its course are different in each individual. What works for one may not work the same, as well, or at all, for another.

Again, the aim of initiating medication therapy is to gain control over inflammation, reduce joint pain and stiffness, and delay disease progression in an effort to give the person with RA the best quality of life possible while research into more effective and safer therapies continues.

OBSTACLES TO GETTING AN EARLY START
Delayed Diagnosis

We explained in Chapter 2 how RA can be difficult to diagnose, especially in its earliest stages. Often the signs and symptoms of the disease are uncharacteristic, the rheumatoid factor test is negative in laboratory tests, or the frontline physician (usually the general practitioner) is unfamiliar with the signs of RA. Whatever the reason, the bottom line is this: Delayed diagnosis results in delayed treatment, and delayed treatment eventually results in irreversible damage to joints.

If you are experiencing unexplained joint pain or prolonged stiffness, or if you have one or more swollen joints, do not rest until you know the cause of it. These symptoms and signs are not part of a "normal health state," and your concern is very real. If your family physician cannot explain the nature of your present condition or suspects you have RA, ask for a referral to a rheumatologist immediately. If you feel your present physician is not hearing your concern, seek a second opinion.

Concern Over Side Effects

If concern over side effects is holding you back from starting (or continuing) medication therapy, you are not alone: In fact, far from it.

A 1999 study that looked at the needs of people with arthritis reported that almost 80 percent were concerned about future side effects from medication therapies.[7] Individuals living with other chronic diseases, like cancer, echo this concern. A 1998 survey looking at patient-centered issues about pain control reported that concerns about side effects was a major barrier to effective treatment.[8]

Whether you will experience side effects from a particular medication therapy will be unknown to you and your rheumatologist ahead of time. However, one thing is certain: Each person will have a different experience, depending on their genetic makeup, past and present health status, and lifestyle. Some individuals may experience minor side effects, and a very few may experience serious side effects. The vast majority experience no side effects at all.

Of greatest importance to you is that in all but the very rare cases, side effects from DMARDs are reversible and, often, may not require stopping the therapy. Side effects like skin reactions, headaches, and dizziness, among others, are common, and are usually managed by the rheumatologist in two ways:

- reduce the dose until the side effect is gone, gradually increasing it back up to the desired dose
- discontinue the therapy and reintroduce it once the side effect subsides

If the side effect returns in either of the above two scenarios, the therapy is usually stopped permanently. At this point, you should discuss the merits of another DMARD and begin taking it as soon as you feel comfortable.

If concern over side effects is present for you, here are some steps you can take to address the issue:

- share your concern about possible side effects with your rheumatologist
- make a list of questions to ask your physician about possible side effects from the medication therapy you are considering
- with the help of your health care team, decide how much risk you are willing to accept in order to gain the benefit from the medication therapy or therapies being considered
- in consultation with your rheumatologist, make a list of goals for each medication therapy being considered, taking into account the severity and prognosis of your RA, your health history, your lifestyle and belief system, and your "comfort zone" for risk
- compare your list of goals against a list of the therapy's known benefits; if few or none of the goals on your list can be met by the benefits of the therapy being considered, the two of you may want to consider another therapy
- before starting medication therapy, ensure that regular monitoring for side effects is available while taking the therapy (e.g., blood and urine tests, regular visits to your rheumatologist, etc.)
- if you have doubts, ask your rheumatologist if they can connect you with others taking the therapy under consideration—the opportunity to speak with someone who has firsthand experience can often prove valuable
- learn all you can about the known benefits, as well as the risks, of each medication therapy being considered

While it is important to know that side effects may occur with any medication, it is even more important for you to know that deformity, disability, and in the worst cases, premature death, will occur if RA is not well controlled. Thus, the benefits of controlling RA are considerable and lifelong.

Also, when looking through reference books on medication, keep in mind that these sources will list *every side effect ever reported, even if it affected only a single individual worldwide.* In fact, even a widely used medication therapy such as acetaminophen (Tylenol® and others) may seem dangerous when one reads the "fine print." Any drug can bring risk, but there is greater risk for the person with RA if medications are avoided.

YOUR MEDICATION THERAPY PLAN

Whether you are diagnosed with mild, moderate, or aggressive RA, medication therapy can play a vital role in your treatment plan. Learning about the known benefits each medication offers, how it is administered and monitored, whether it suits your lifestyle, and its possible side effects will help you make choices you can live with over the short and long terms.

Get Expert Advice

Medication recommendations should come from a rheumatologist with ample experience prescribing both approved and experimental RA medications. Although your GP (if you have one) may oversee blood, urine, and other safety monitoring tests, they rarely prescribe aggressive medication therapy early on for RA. In fact, a study published in a leading medical journal reported that while 73 percent of GPs were aware of DMARDs and knew their value, only 14 percent prescribed them to their patients.[9]

Administering the correct DMARD, and doing so in a manner that maximizes benefits and minimizes risks, requires considerable experience. Combination DMARD therapy requires even more skill. Physicians who lack experience with DMARDs may use too low a dose or give up on the therapy too early; they may not know how to recognize or reduce side effects; and they may fail to use other medication therapies while waiting for a DMARD to start working. Worst of all, they may not start you on a DMARD at all.

In remote areas of some countries, a rheumatologist may not be easily available. Hopefully, there will be an internist with arthritis training who serves as a part-time rheumatologist. As a rule of thumb, a physician, even a rheumatologist, who is not working with more than one hundred individuals with RA would not be highly experienced. When the rheumatologist is not your primary care physician (this is true outside of the United States), the family physician can play an important role. He or she can help to monitor for medication side effects; address other general health issues (e.g., flu shots and preventative checkups) and concerns (e.g., osteoporosis, high cholesterol), and help coordinate other specialists required (e.g., orthopedic surgeon, physiotherapist, occupational therapist, ophthalmologist).

Gather Information

First and foremost, know all you can about the medication therapies being recommended. Try to get a range of information, from the very basic to the very technical. Easy-to-understand information about RA therapies can often be obtained from voluntary health organizations such as the Arthritis Foundation (United States and Australia), the Arthritis Society (Canada), Arthritis Care (United Kingdom), and the Arthritis Foundation of New Zealand (Inc.). Reliable, "user-friendly" information also can be found on the Internet, at the public library, or at university based bookstores. (See Chapter 12 for additional information available to you.)

If your disease prevents or limits you from gathering the information you need to make informed decisions, ask family members and friends to give you a hand. This provides them with a terrific opportunity to learn about your disease and feel like they are providing you with wanted support, while saving you precious energy.

Ask Questions

Prepare a list of questions (make several copies) to ask your rheumatologist about the recommended medications. Make every effort to be well organized: They may have limited time available to answer questions. If that is the case, prioritize your questions and ask those that are most important to you during the actual office visit. Leave a written copy of the list with your rheumatologist so that a follow-up note or phone call can cover your remaining questions—preferably within a week's time.

Here is a sample list of questions to help get you started:

- How long has the recommended medication been in use?
- How will I take the medication? By mouth, needle, intravenously?
- What is the standard dosage?
- What are the known benefits?
- What are the known potential side effects?
- If I experience side effects, are they reversible (or permanent) when the medication is stopped?
- If I stop the medication, how long will it stay in my body?
- Is the recommended medication, proven effective against disease severity comparable to mine?
- When will I start to get better?
- Can I reduce the dose once I get better?
- How long will the medication work?
- Can I take the medication if I am attempting to conceive a baby? (for women and men)
- Can I take the medication if I am pregnant?
- Can I take the medication if I am breast-feeding?
- If I take the medication, will it prevent me from ever having children? (for women and men)

Monitor for Safety

Make sure to ask your rheumatologist or pharmacist for detailed written instructions on dosage, information on possible side effects, and blood and urine monitoring procedures (if these are required) before you start taking the therapy. The information should be presented in a way that is easy to understand. If not, ask your rheumatologist to explain anything that remains unclear before you start the therapy.

Many DMARD therapies are initiated in incremental doses over several weeks or months. Think of these first few weeks as a "test dose phase" designed to test your tolerance for the therapy and to look for signs of possible side effects. If you tolerate the therapy and show no signs of side effects, the dose will be increased to the full treatment dose or to the level that leads to maximal improvement in your RA. The latter is sometimes called the *maintenance dose.*

If you develop side effects or have difficulty tolerating a DMARD, it is sometimes possible to lower the dose with a disappearance of the side effects but continuing benefit, or your doctor may increase the dose again without the side effect reappearing. Because DMARDs are the key to controlling RA, it is imperative that the person guiding your treatment is both expert and highly experienced in the use of these medications.

For most DMARDs, from the time you start taking the medication to the time you stop, your blood and urine (and possibly other factors, depending on the medication used) should be tested for signs of side effects. These tests detect abnormalities that are not physically apparent to your physician during office examinations. Detecting abnormalities early is the key to preventing serious side effects. In addition, ophthalmologic (eye) exams or bone density tests may be required periodically when taking specific medications (hydroxychlorquine and prednisone, respectively).

Table 4.1 lists lab tests commonly required when taking RA medications. Becoming well-versed with test names and meanings (including their short forms or acronyms) will help you monitor your health along with your physician. The column titled "normal values" may vary with the specific laboratory; ask the laboratory processing your tests for their "normal values" chart.

If one of your lab tests does happen to come back slightly below or above the "normal value" range, this may not be cause for concern. Why? Because if one hundred healthy people walked into a lab to be tested, for any one test performed, five would have a test result that would fall slightly outside of the "normal value." That is how "normal" is defined in a medical laboratory. Another way to think of it is that if your doctor ordered a battery of twenty tests, one could come back slightly out of the "normal value" range, but still be normal.

The hematocrit, hemoglobin, red blood cell count, white blood cell count, and platelet count, as well as other measures on the red blood cells, are called the *complete blood count,* or "CBC."

Table 4.1 lists some of the more common tests your physician may order. However, depending on disease severity and duration, and depending on your customized medication therapy regime, your physician may order tests not listed above. For additional information on specific tests required for specific medication therapies, please refer to the Evidence-Based Medications section in this chapter.

TABLE 4.1. COMMON RA LAB TESTS

Test Name & Type	Normal Values	Unit of Measure	Test Description
BLOOD TESTS			
Hematocrit (HCT)	Women 0.35–0.46 Men 0.41–0.50	liter per liter	These two tests measure the amount of hemoglobin (the oxygen-carrying protein) in your blood. Low counts may signal a possible blood loss from your stomach, or may be a sign you are producing fewer red blood cells. The latter is common when RA is active but can occur rarely due to medication therapy.
Hemoglobin (Hgb)	Women 120–150 Men 133–165	grams per liter	
Red Blood Cell Count (RBC)	Women 3.80–4.80 Men 4.2–5.40	tera per liter	Measures the number of red blood cells in your system. The red blood cells carry hemoglobin and this test is related to the hemoglobin and hematocrit.
White Blood Cell Count (WBC)	Women 4.0–10.0 Men 4.0–10.0	giga per liter	Measures the number of white blood cells in your blood. The number can increase with infection or use of prednisone. A decreased number can result from medication therapy, and rarely, from RA. A very low number (<1) would increase your chances of developing an infection.
Platelet Count	Women & Men 150–350	giga per liter	Platelets help blood to clot. If your number of platelets is extremely low, you may bruise easily and bleeding can become difficult to stop. This can occur with Felty's syndrome (a variety of RA), or due to medications.

Test	Sex	Range	Units	Description
				The platelet count also may be increased in RA, usually when the disease is very active.
Erythrocyte Sedimentation Rate (ESR)	Women Men	0–20 0–10	millimeter per hour	Commonly called "sed rate" (for sedimentation), this test value rises with increased inflammation from arthritis or other conditions such as major infections. The higher your "sed rate," the greater the amount of inflammation. This number will likely go down if your medication therapy is effective.
C-Reactive Protein (CRP)	Women & Men	<5	milligrams per liter	This test is another, more expensive, measure of inflammation. It is used more commonly in Europe than in North America.
Albumin (Protein)	Women & Men	35–50	grams per liter	This test measures a major blood protein. Many medication therapies bind to the protein. Very low levels may increase the effect of some medications such as methotrexate.
Salicylate	Women & Men	150–250	milligrams per liter	Salicylate is the active ingredient in aspirin (taken to reduce inflammation). This test tells you how much salicylate your body is absorbing; too high a level can be harmful.

LIVER FUNCTION TESTS

Test	Sex	Range	Units	Description
Aspartate Aminotransferase (AST)	Women & Men	10–40	units per liter	Liver function tests are often called "LFTs." Used to monitor toxicity in your liver from medication therapies such as methotrexate, azathioprine, or NSAIDS. The gamma GT is another test sometimes used to monitor liver function.
Alanine Aminotransferase (ALT)	Women & Men	10–60		

	Women & Men varies with technique used	
Alkaline Phosphatase ("Alk Phos")		
Creatinine	micromole per liter	This test measures how well your kidney is functioning. Creatinine is a normal waste product of muscle; when found in too high a level, it indicates that your kidney is not working well enough to clear waste products from your body. While the blood test is accurate, your physician may occasionally need a collection of urine over twenty four hours for a very precise measure of kidney function.

	Women 50–100 Men 70–120	

OTHER TESTS

Urine Test	N/A	A "urinalysis" detects the presence of protein, red or white blood cells, or other abnormalities in your urine. A "dipstick" is a strip which when immersed in urine will measure protein and red and white blood cells; it is a simple and inexpensive test. A more detailed test includes a microscopic examination of the urine to actually count the number of red and white blood cells. For a very accurate measure of protein, you will have to collect your urine for twenty four hours. Regular monitoring of the urine is required when taking D-penicillamine and gold therapy.
Stool Guaiac		This test detects blood in the bowel movement not noticeable on visual examination. This can be a sign of "silent" bleeding from NSAIDs.
Joint Fluid Test	<0.2 giga/L	This test analyzes synovial fluid from a specific joint(s). It can determine the extent of the inflammation and is the definitive test to exclude an infection in a joint or diagnose an accompanying case of gout or

pseudogout. A white blood cell count can be determined on synovial fluid. A level of greater than 2 is found in inflammatory conditions such as RA.

Biopsy Tests	Tissue removed and examined microscopically to detect damage or to establish diagnosis. Biopsies of the skin, muscle, liver, lung, or synovium (the lining of the joint) are among the most common.		
X-rays	X-rays detect early damage to joints. Subsequent x-rays assess whether the disease is progressing. X-rays are most commonly taken of smaller joints like those in the hands and feet, as this is where damage is usually first detected.	N/A	N/A
Vision Tests	If you are taking hydroxychloroquine and your eyes were healthy before beginning the medication, special vision tests—usually performed by an ophthalmologist (eye doctor)—are done about every twelve to eighteen months to detect the earliest sign of side effects and avert permanent damage. Some individuals may require testing more frequently.	Vary by test	Vary by test

Stick With It

Earlier in this chapter, we explained that a common reason individuals abandon DMARD therapy is because they fear the potential side effects. Another common reason is, of course, simply not taking the medication. One study of people with RA showed that 22 percent reported to their physicians that they were not taking their prescribed medication, 60 percent were not following their exercise plan, and 75 percent were not wearing their splints.[10, 11] Why? The reasons vary: Research tells us that a certain percentage doubt the therapy will work; another group does not understand the way in which the therapy should work; and still others do not take the medication if they need to take it several times a day.[12]

If you want to benefit from the medication being prescribed but are having difficulty sticking with it, there are some simple steps you can take to increase your chances for success significantly. The single most important step to take is to develop a strong relationship with your rheumatologist. The strength of this relationship greatly influences your willingness to stick with your medication.[13] Share your concerns about potential side effects with your rheumatologist, and ask questions about the medications recommended. Interestingly, those who do ask questions about the medication being recommended are viewed more positively by their physicians; the physician considers these individuals more interested and assertive.[14]

Other steps you can take to stick with it are:

- Reach agreement with your rheumatologist on your diagnosis: If you do not believe the diagnosis, chances are you will not believe in the medication. Because this is so important to the success of your treatment, if you are unable to reach agreement, seek a second opinion (the opinion of another expert). Your rheumatologist will welcome it, because he or she wants you to feel certain of your diagnosis. The same is true for the treatment. If you are not convinced that the medication being recommended is for you, get a second opinion. It may cost you some time and money, but knowing you are on the right track is paramount.
- Understand the health risks of not treating your disease with effective therapies: For all individuals with RA, the risk of long-term disability and even premature death is substantially greater than the risk of serious side effects from medication therapy.
- Understand the goals of your medication therapy: What are the benefits (e.g., reduced inflammation, less pain, greater mobility, etc.)? If you don't know what to expect from your medication therapy, it will be difficult to assess its short- or long-term effectiveness.

- With the help of your rheumatologist, create a dosing schedule that works with your pattern of daily activities.
- Post a calendar in an obvious place reminding you of your prescribed dosing schedule.
- Use a clearly labeled medication organizer to keep medications separated by type and day. You can usually find them at your local pharmacy.
- Follow the blood and urine monitoring schedule recommended by your rheumatologist to ensure safety.
- Ask family members and friends to be supportive of your medication therapy decisions and plans.

Evaluate the Results

Evaluating the results of each of your medications is important, and should guide you and your rheumatologist in making decisions about when to increase or decrease the dosage—or discontinue it altogether. First, you must know what to expect from each of the medications in your plan. This is particularly true for DMARDs. Each one takes a different length of time to reach its full therapeutic potential.

For example, a person on methotrexate may only need to wait a month or two to see results, while gold salts may take twice as long. It may be necessary to add another DMARD to the methotrexate to maximize its benefit. Regardless, whenever a new DMARD (or any other medication or treatment therapy) is included into your overall plan, begin monitoring the changes you notice using your health journal.

The following self-evaluation chart will help you track how you feel over time during your treatment. On a scale of 1 to 10 (where 1 is "agree totally" and 10 is "totally disagree"), rate each of the following five statements:

1. Joint pain and stiffness are severe first thing in the morning.
   1 2 3 4 5 6 7 8 9 10
2. Self-care activities such as showering, hair combing, and getting dressed are painful and difficult.   1 2 3 4 5 6 7 8 9 10
3. Daily activities such as walking, climbing stairs, standing to sitting (and vice versa), driving, and so on are painful and difficult.
   1 2 3 4 5 6 7 8 9 10
4. Daily activities like working outside of the home, carrying groceries, preparing meals, housework, gardening, are painful and difficult.   1 2 3 4 5 6 7 8 9 10
5. Recreational activities such as gardening, bicycling, weight-bearing exercise, or other weight-bearing activities are painful and difficult.   1 2 3 4 5 6 7 8 9 10

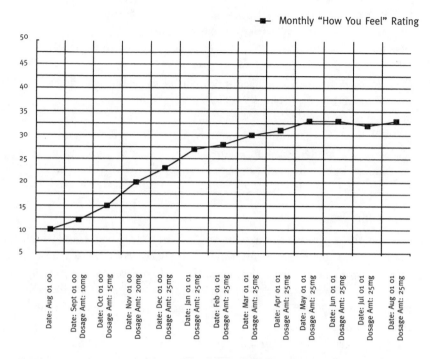

Fig. 4.1. "How You Feel" Self-evaluation Chart. The worst you have felt = 5, the best you have felt = 50.

Add up your score—out of a possible fifty points—and then chart the number in the appropriate column. Remember, in order for this self-evaluation chart to be meaningful to you, and relevant to your physician, it is important to rate "how you feel" from the start of the new medication, at regular one-month intervals, and each time the dosage is increased or decreased. If you are diligent in recording this information, you should see an improving trend, a leveling-off, or a downward trend in the months following the start of the medication.

Figure 4.1 depicts a sample "How You Feel" Self-evaluation Chart of a person taking methotrexate therapy over a twelve-month period. At the start date, the person rated herself at ten, a low score, indicating that she was having a fair degree of difficulty managing most of the items listed in the chart. However, you can see that, over time, she began to feel significantly better, achieving an overall rating of thirty-three at the end of twelve months of therapy.

EVIDENCE-BASED MEDICATIONS

For persons with RA, understanding the difference between therapies proven effective and those that have not is critical to the success of their treatment plan. Why? Time.

As discussed earlier, joint damage from RA starts early—probably within weeks after disease symptoms appear. Particularly for the 30 to 70 percent of individuals diagnosed with moderate to aggressive RA, one can ill afford to spend months or years experimenting with unproven therapies. Whether the therapy recommended to you is medication therapy, naturopathic therapy, physical therapy, or vitamin therapy, make certain there is solid research proving its effectiveness.

The bottom line is this: Swollen, inflamed joints mean the disease is not controlled. Damage to your joint and the adjacent bone, tendons, and ligaments will be the result of ineffective and unproven therapies.

Ask for the Evidence

A medication "proven effective" receives government approval for use in the broad population after undergoing rigorous scientific study (publication of these studies in reputable medical journals is your "evidence"). Usually, the first studies of an experimental medication are short term, up to one year. The results of these studies prove—or disprove—the effectiveness of the medication, as well as report the frequency and type of side effects experienced by study participants (people with RA). The results of these research studies provide physicians the scientific information they need to make appropriate recommendations about medication. Medications in use for decades continue to be studied to identify new uses and to help researchers and physicians further refine practice guidelines for health professionals treating people with RA.

It is important for you to know that while medications described in this section are proven effective, no one medication will produce the same results in any two individuals. To use the snowflake analogy again, the course of RA is unique in every individual and requires an individualized medication therapy plan.

Medications Proven Effective

RA medications proven effective fall into two categories: NSAIDs and DMARDs. However, as discussed earlier in this chapter, research and best treatment practice today show that DMARDs are the key to achieving better long-term results. To simplify the terminology, we place proven medications into two easy to understand and remember categories:

1. Symptom Management Medication (SMM)
2. Disease Management Medication (DMM)

One potentially confusing aspect of medications is that every drug has at least two names. Every company that makes a drug gives it a brand name. Not surprisingly, different companies use different brand names. Sometimes one drug from a single company will have different brand names in different countries—something that may cause confusion if you are travel-ing and run out of your medication. The second name that every medica-tion has is the generic name which is the chemical name and is the same worldwide. By convention, the generic name is not capitalized and the brand name is. For example, ibuprofen is the generic name for an over-the-counter anti-inflammatory, and Motrin® and Advil® are two of the many brand names used to market ibuprofen by different companies.

SYMPTOM MANAGEMENT MEDICATION (SMM)

SMMs include *analgesics* and *nonsteroidal anti-inflammatory drugs* (NSAIDs). See Table 4.2 for a list of the more commonly used and pre-scribed SMMs. Typically, physicians will prescribe SMMs at the first signs of inflammation, often before they or a rheumatologist confirms a diagno-sis of RA. You may have to try several different SMMs to find the one that is most effective in managing the symptoms, and most easily tolerated by your body. Analgesics are pain relievers. They do nothing to limit inflam-mation. Acetaminophen is an inexpensive and safe pain reliever. Your physician may suggest you use it along with your other medications. Codeine, a pain reliever in the narcotic class, is also an analgesic. Codeine is commonly combined with acetaminophen. Because codeine is a mild nar-cotic, it has side effects, such as making you sleepy and constipated. In addi-tion to being potentially habit-forming, they do not slow down the RA, so most rheumatologists are against the frequent- or regular-use of pain re-lievers containing codeine or other narcotics.

NSAIDs

In contrast to analgesics, NSAIDs do reduce the effects of the inflamma-tion, especially stiffness and pain. They do not deal with the underlying RA process that causes the inflammation, however. So, NSAIDs can make you feel better, but don't limit or stop the process that damages the joints. Most people with RA need to take NSAIDs.

While some NSAIDs are sufficiently safe for governments to approve over-the-counter sale, that does not mean they are free of side effects. Both over-the-counter and prescription NSAIDs have side effects. Side effects are more common at higher doses and people with RA tend to need these higher doses to control the inflammation caused by the disease. When one considers full doses of traditional NSAIDs, the frequency of side effects tends to be the same, on average, for all the different medications. Thus, you and your physician will often choose the NSAID that you tolerate the best and from which you get the most benefit.

The most common side effects of *traditional NSAIDs* (see Table 4.2 for a list) involve the stomach. These are: gastric irritation (GI) and ulcers. An ulcer is like a crater in the stomach; a small ulcer is called an erosion.

In the United States, the chance of hospitalization due to a GI side effect from an NSAID is 1.3 to 1.6 percent over the course of twelve months, or 1 in 3 people with RA over the entire course of the person's disease.[15] A recent study conducted in Europe concluded that, on average, 1 in 1,200 individuals taking a traditional NSAID for at least two months will die from stomach complications, but would not have died had they not been taking the medication.[16] You can see why rheumatologists now consider the Disease Management Medications (discussed below) to be relatively safe.

Your risk of experiencing traditional NSAID-related side effects is increased if you:

- have RA
- are sixty-five-plus years of age
- are taking aspirin (many seniors take baby aspirin to reduce the risk of heart disease and stroke)
- are taking anticoagulants (blood thinners)
- are using corticosteroids (such as prednisone)
- had a previous peptic (stomach) ulcer or bleeding thought to be due to an ulcer
- have other illnesses or conditions such as heart, liver, or kidney disease
- are taking a maximal dose of a traditional NSAID.[17]

This list of "predictors" for serious stomach problems is helpful. Unfortunately, it does not help to identify everyone likely to have a bad result from traditional NSAIDs. A study conducted at Stanford University showed that a large majority of people with RA on traditional NSAID therapy who then developed serious gastro-intestinal complications *did not have preceding side effects—not even mild ones.*[18] In essence, this study was the first of many to show that the person with RA taking traditional NSAID therapy was taking an extreme risk with their stomach.

For those with one or more of the predictors in the above list, there are some medications that, when taken along with traditional NSAIDs, can reduce the risk of developing an ulcer, especially a bad one that bleeds or perforates (literally, makes a hole through the stomach wall). One group of these medications is called *proton pump inhibitors.* These reduce the stomach's production of acid. Common proton pump inhibitors include omeprazole (Prilosec®, Losec®) and iansoprazole (Prevacid®). Another medication called misoprostol (Cytotec®) replaces the stomach-protecting prostaglandin molecules that are consumed by the traditional NSAIDs. However, adding one of these medications can cause additional side effects to those of traditional NSAIDs. For instance, about one in four people

TABLE 4.2. SYMPTOM MANAGEMENT MEDICATIONS

Generic Medication Name (Brand Name)	Use/Benefit	Adult Dose Range	How Long Before It Works	Safety Monitoring Tests	Side Effects, Cautions
OVER-THE-COUNTER					
aspirin or ASA (acetylated salicylates) (Anacin®, Bayer®, Bufferin®, Excedrin®, etc.)	Used to treat against inflammation. Because of the risk of ulcers, only "enteric-coated" aspirin should be taken long-term. Also, because aspirin overdose can occur easily, a physician should be involved in adjusting the dose at the high levels used to treat RA.	1300–4000 mg. per day in three or four doses daily. Always take with food. Taken by mouth.	Should see benefit on pain and stiffness within two weeks' time.	A blood aspirin level can be measured to determine if nonresponse to the therapy is due to too low a level or if the blood level is too high.	*Possible side effects include:* Abdominal cramps and pain, gastric ulcers, heartburn or indigestion, nausea or vomiting, ringing in the ears, deafness, tendency for increased bleeding. *Use caution or avoid use if you:* Are sensitive or allergic to aspirin or nonacetylated salicylates; have kidney, liver disease, or heart disease; have high blood pressure, asthma, peptic ulcers, or use anticoagulants. Do not take acetylated salicylates while taking NSAIDs unless directed by your rheumatologist.

Drug	Uses	Dosage	Benefit	Possible side effects
Nonacetylated salicylates *magnesium choline salicylate* *salsalate* *sodium salicylate*	Used to treat against inflammation. May have less gastrointestinal (stomach) side effects than aspirin.	Varies by brand. See packaging for dosing instructions. Always take with food. Taken by mouth. 1500–4000 mg/day 1500–5000 mg/day 3000–5000 mg/day	Should see benefit on pain and stiffness within two weeks' time.	*Possible side effects include:* If you use alcohol, chances of gastric ulcers and bleeding, as well as kidney and liver damage, are increased. Side effects may be more pronounced for people with preexisting heart or kidney disease. May cause confusion in the elderly and people with kidney impairment.
acetaminophen (Tylenol®, Panadol®, Aspirin Free Anacin®, etc)	Used to relieve pain symptoms; acetaminophen has no effect against inflammation.	1000–4000 mg/day in three to four doses daily. Always take with food. Taken by mouth.	Should see benefit on pain, usually within thirty minutes.	*Possible side effects include:* If you use alcohol excessively, fast, or take excessive amounts of acetaminophen, may damage the kidney or liver. *Use caution or avoid use if you:* Have a history of alcohol abuse, kidney disease, hepatitis, or other liver disease.

Generic Medication Name (Brand Name)	Use/Benefit	Adult Dose Range	How Long Before It Works	Safety Monitoring Test	Side Effects, Cautions
PRESCRIPTION					
Traditional NSAIDs Listed below are some of the more commonly prescribed brands	Used to treat more aggressive or chronic inflammation of the joint(s) and resulting stiffness and pain.	Dosage varies depending on the brand. Always take with food to protect the lining of the stomach. Taken by mouth.	Should see benefit on pain and stiffness within two weeks' time.	*On starting:* CBC, creatinine (first three weeks if you are also taking an "ACE" inhibitor, beta blocker, or diuretic), AST and ALT (within eight weeks after starting).	*Possible side effects include:* Dizziness, drowsiness, nausea, fatigue or weakness, vomiting, ringing in ears, rash, greater susceptibility to bruising or bleeding, abdominal pain, diarrhea, gastric ulcers and bleeding, heartburn, indigestion, nightmares, fluid retention.
diclofenac (Voltaren®) fenoprofen (Nalfon®) flurbiprofen (Ansaid®) ibuprofen (Motrin®) indomethacin (Indocin®) ketoprofen (Orudis®) meclofenamate (Meclomen®) meloxicam (Mobic®) nabumetone (Relafen®) naproxen (Naprosyn®) piroxicam (Feldene®) sulindac (Clinoril®) tolmetin (Tolectin®)		100–150 mg/day 1200–3200 mg/day 100–300 mg/day 1200–3200 mg/day 50–200 mg/day 150–300 mg/day 200–400 mg/day 7.5–15 mg/day 1000–2000 mg/day 500–1500 mg/day 10–20 mg/day 300–400 mg/day 1200–1800 mg/day		*Annually:* CBC, LFTs, creatinine.	*Use caution or avoid use if you:* Are sensitive or allergic to aspirin, nonacetylated salicylates, or similar medications; have kidney or liver disease; have heart disease; have high blood pressure; asthma; peptic ulcers; take anticoagulants. Do not take aspirin while taking NSAIDs unless directed by your rheumatologist.

COX-2 selective NSAIDs	Used to treat against inflammation of the joint(s) and resulting stiffness and pain. Major advantage of these therapies is reduced frequency of ulcers and stomach bleeding. Probably safer if you have to take a blood thinner, such as warfarin.	Always take with food. Taken by mouth.	You should see full benefit within two weeks after you start taking it.	*On starting:* CBC, creatinine (first three weeks if you are also taking an "ace" inhibitor or diuretic), AST and ALT (within 8 weeks after starting). *Annually:* CBC, LFTs, creatinine.	*Possible side effects include:* Dizziness, drowsiness, nausea, fatigue or weakness, vomiting, ringing in ears, rash, greater susceptibility to bruising or bleeding, abdominal pain, gastric ulcers and bleeding, heartburn, indigestion, nightmares, hypertension, fluid retention). *Use caution or avoid use if you:* Are elderly, frail, or debilitated, or if you seem to experience more frequent or more severe side effects.
celecoxib (Celebrex®)		200–400 mg per day			If you are allergic to sulfa-based antibiotics you should not take celecoxib without specific permission and instruction from your physician.
rofecoxib (Vioxx®)		12.5–25 mg per day			Rofecoxib may increase the blood level of methotrexate. It may increase the chance of heart attack in high risk individuals.

started on a full dose of misoprostol develop intolerable diarrhea, abdominal cramps, or feel bloated.

In 1999, the risk of developing serious GI complications was substantially reduced with the development and approval of a new class of NSAIDs, called *COX-2 selective NSAIDs*. Scientists discovered that the traditional NSAID worked by blocking a protein which existed in two forms, COX-1 and COX-2. They learned that blocking the COX-1 protein led to stomach irritation and ulcers, as well as affected the platelets (small blood cells that are sticky and help clotting), and that blocking the COX-2 protein delivered the desired anti-inflammatory effects. Thus, the new COX-2 selective NSAIDs reduce the risk of a serious ulcer, bleeding, or a perforation (a hole in the stomach) by about 50 percent. However, the COX-2 selective NSAIDs do not protect against heart attacks, like aspirin does, and low-dose aspirin may have to be taken by some, limiting the GI protection of the Cox-2 selective drug.

The bottom line on NSAID medications, is this: If you want the least amount of GI risk, ask your rheumatologist to prescribe a COX-2 selective NSAID. However, be prepared to pay more. Because COX-2 selective NSAIDs are newer and protected by patents, they are more expensive than traditional NSAIDs, many of which are available as generic medications.

Whether you are taking a traditional NSAID or a COX-2 selective NSAID, it is best to take them with food. If you develop persistent heartburn, hunger pains, or other abdominal (tummy) pain, call your doctor and let him or her know. If your bowel movements become jet black in color, a possible sign of stomach bleeding, call your doctor immediately. (Be aware that iron supplements also make bowel movements black in color.)

In that NSAIDs don't stop RA, take the amount you need to suppress the pain and stiffness. In other words, don't skimp and suffer, but don't take more than you need.

The traditional NSAIDs affect the platelets and reduce their ability to function as well as normal. Aspirin does this the best of all, which is the reason small doses of aspirin are used to prevent heart disease and stroke. The platelet effect enhances bleeding due to stomach ulcers. The COX-2 selective NSAIDs do not have this effect on platelets, and thus are the NSAID of choice when an anticoagulant (blood thinner) must be taken, too. In general, an NSAID should not be taken with an anticoagulant, but if an NSAID is absolutely necessary, a COX-2 selective NSAID is probably safer. While the lack of platelet effect may be a benefit, it is also potentially a problem. The traditional NSAID's effects on the platelets may protect somewhat against heart attack and stroke. If an individual is changing to a COX-2 agent, they should first discuss it with their rheumatologist or family doctor.

Other common side effects of traditional and COX-2 selective NSAIDs include: allergy (as it is with almost all medication therapies); hives and other skin rashes; ringing in the ears (aspirin); and headache (indomethacin). Some with RA find that one NSAID leaves them feeling less alert or even confused, but another will be well tolerated.

Both traditional and COX-2 selective NSAIDs can interfere with the effectiveness of medications to control high blood pressure. For individuals taking both NSAIDs and high blood pressure medication, the blood pressure should be checked several times after starting the NSAID.

All of the NSAIDs (traditional and COX-2 selective) can, on rare occasions, affect the kidney or liver. Kidney effects may be more common with the traditional NSAIDs indomethacin and fenoprofen. Liver test abnormalities are most frequent with diclofenac, another traditional NSAID.

Other rare side effects of traditional and COX-2 selective NSAIDs are major reductions in the body's ability to make red or white blood cells.

DISEASE MANAGEMENT MEDICATION (DMM)

See table 4.3 for a list of commonly prescribed DMMs. Designed to control the disease itself, this group of medication is one of the most important aspects of your treatment plan. Each one works against RA in a different way, and may be used in combination against more aggressive or severe RA. When DMMs are effective, they control the disease process. How will you know if they are working? When the disease is well controlled, you should experience less joint stiffness, less joint pain, less fatigue, and greater strength and mobility. Most important, your joints will become less swollen. Your rheumatologist or GP will monitor blood tests to confirm the improvement; the ESR is the most commonly monitored.

Most DMMs take anywhere from three to twelve weeks to begin working; some take even longer. If the DMM prescribed to you is effective, you should notice subtle improvements at first: less stiffness in the morning or after sitting for extended periods, less joint pain, less fatigue, and greater ability to perform activities of daily living such as washing, dressing, and preparing meals. While the timing will differ depending on the DMM, if you see little or no improvement within the first six weeks to three months after beginning the medication, discuss the benefits and risks of increasing the dosage amount with your rheumatologist, or discuss adding another to form a combination therapy.

A general approach to DMMs

There are no hard and fast rules as to how best to use DMMs in any one person with RA. What follows is a "sketch" plan.

Mild RA. For mild RA, many rheumatologists would use hydroxy-chloroquine, sulfasalazine, minocycline, or oral gold. Minocycline

TABLE 4.3. PRESCRIPTION DISEASE MANAGEMENT MEDICATIONS

Generic Medication Name (Brand Name)	Use/Benefit	Average Adult Maintenance Dose Range	How Long Before It Works	Monitoring Tests	Side Effects, Cautions
azathioprine (Imuran®)	Used to treat severe RA by suppressing the immune system. Although this therapy can be effective in treatment of RA, it is more toxic than other RA medication therapies and thus reserved for severe RA.	50 to 200 mg. per day in one to three doses, based on body weight Take with food. Taken by mouth.	If effective, benefits are seen within eight to twelve weeks.	*On starting:* CBC, platelet count, creatinine, AST or ALT. *Ongoing:* CBC and platelet count every one to two weeks when dosage is changed, and every one to three months thereafter.	*Possible side effects include:* Loss of appetite, nausea or vomiting, skin rash, bone marrow suppression, infection, malignancy, pancreatitis. *Use caution or avoid use if you:* Have or had kidney or liver disease; are currently using allopurinol (a medication for gout).
cyclophosphamide (Cytoxan®)	Used to treat vasculitis or inflammation of the blood vessels due to RA by suppressing the immune system. This is a highly effective but toxic RA medication, generally reserved for very	Up to 1000 mg/m² (m² is a measure of the body surface area). Taken intravenously (into a vein by needle).	If effective, benefits are seen in seven to ten days.	*On starting:* CBC, platelet count, creatinine, AST or ALT. *Ongoing:* CBC and platelet count every one to two weeks when dosage is	*Possible side effects include:* Infertility in men and women; loss of appetite; bone marrow suppression; infection; bleeding from the bladder; cancer. *Use caution or avoid use if you:* Have or had kidney or liver disease; have an active infection; are pregnant.

| cyclosporine-A (Neoral®) | severe disease. Often, there is limited or no other option left when this therapy is required.

Cyclosporine is generally used in those individuals with moderate to severe RA not responding to other DMMs. | Benefit is typically seen within eight to twelve weeks.

2.5–5.0 mg per kg per day in 1 or 2 doses.

Taken by mouth.

Store in the refrigerator. | changed, and every one to three months thereafter.

On starting: CBC, creatinine, uric acid, LFTs, BP (blood pressure).

Ongoing: Creatinine every two weeks until dose is stable, then monthly. Also, periodic CBC, potassium, and LFTs. | **Do not use during pregnancy.**

Possible side effects include: Bleeding of the gums; tender or enlarged gums; fluid retention; hypertension; increase in hair growth; decreased kidney function; loss of appetite; trembling or shaking of hands; numbness.

Rare side effects include: Suppression of ability to make blood cells; liver toxicity and increased infections. Very rarely, lymph gland cancer can occur.

Use caution or avoid use if you: Are sensitive to castor oil (if taking drug by injection); have liver or kidney disease; have an active infection; have hypertension. |

Generic Medication Name (Brand Name)	Use/Benefit	Average Adult Maintenance Dose Range	How Long Before It Works	Monitoring Tests	Side Effects, Cautions
etanercept (Enbrel®)	One of the new "anti-TNF" RA medicationtherapies. Because of its higher cost, it ispresently being given to those with moderate to severe RA or those not responding to other DMMs.	25 mg twice weekly. Taken by injection under the skin.	Benefit is typically seen within two weeks.	Not required.	*Possible side effects include:* Check with your doctor if you experience chills, cough, fever or skin rash, or frequent or painful urination. Injection site reactions are common. The risk of cancer is a potential concern that has has not been confirmed to date. However, long-term studies are pending. The development of autoantibodies is increased. Serious infections, multiple sclerosis–like disorders, and reduced blood counts have occurred and rarely have resulted in death. *Use caution or avoid use if you:* Are pregnant; are breast-feeding; had allergic reaction to Enbrel or any of its components.
gold salt injections *gold sodium thiomalate* (Myochrysine®)	Used to treat mild RA not responding to other DMMs, and moderate to severe RA, sometimes in	25 mg to 50 mg in a single dose weekly. Administered/	Benefits in three to four months, with maximum benefit for some at twelve months.	*On starting:* CBC, creatinine, platelet count; and urine dipstick for protein.	*Possible side effects:* Mouth ulcers and itchy rash are common. Suppression of the ability to make blood cells (red cells, white cells, or platelets) and the development of protein leakage from

Drug	Notes	Dose	Monitoring	Side effects / Cautions
gold thioglucose (Solganol®)	combination with methotrexate or hydroxychloroquine. Gold salts are generally slow-acting, but are highly effective with a good safety record.	Self-administered by deep intramuscular injection.	*Every one to two weeks for first twenty weeks at the time of each (or every other) injection:* CBC; platelet count; urine dipstick. *Ongoing:* creatinine every two weeks until dose is stable, then monthly. Also, periodic CBC and LFTs.	the kidney are rare but potentially serious. Lung and bowel side effects are very rare. *Use caution or avoid use if you:* Have kidney disease, bone marrow suppression, colitis (inflamed bowels).
gold by mouth auranofin (Ridaura®)	Used to treat mild RA. Felt to be the least effective of the drugs for mild RA and much less effective than gold salt injections. Used less and less frequently.	3 mg twice daily. If no benefit by three months, dose is increased to 3 mg three times daily by mouth. Benefits seen over three months. If no benefit by six months, drug is discontinued.	*On starting:* CBC, platelet count, creatinine, urine dipstick for protein. *Ongoing:* CBC, platelet count, urine dipstick for protein monthly for six months, then quarterly.	*Possible side effects:* These are similar to gold salt injections but less common. Diarrhea is more common and occurs in more than 10-percent. *Use caution or avoid use if you:* Have kidney disease, bone marrow suppression, colitis (inflamed bowels).

Generic Medication Therapy Name (Brand Name)	Use/Benefit	Average Adult Maintenance Dose Range	How Long Before It Works	Monitoring Tests	Side Effects, Cautions
hydroxychloroquine sulfate (Plaquenil®)	An antimalarial medication and one of the safest DMMs, primarily used for milder forms of RA or in combination with other DMMs for more aggressive RA. Another antimalarial medication, chloroquine (Aralen®), is used in some parts of the world, but because of increased toxicity on the eye it is not used in North America.	Maximum dose of hydroxy-chloroquine should not exceed 6.5 mg/kg or 3 mg/lb of lean body weight/day in one or two doses daily. *The maximum daily dosage should not exceed 400 mg, even if the person weighs more than 61 kg or 135 lb.* Take with food.	If effective, you should notice an improvement in symptoms within three to six months, although improvement can continue for a year.	*On starting:* None, unless you are over 40 years old or have previous eye disease. *Ongoing:* You should have an eye exam by an ophthamologist (medical doctor eye specialist) within twelve months after the date you started taking the medication and annually thereafter, or more frequently if you have liver or kidney problems, or eye abnormalities.	*Possible side effects:* Diarrhea, loss of appetite, nausea, stomach cramps or pain, skin rash, neuromyopathy. Eye damage and damage to muscles and nerves are very rare. Can affect the blood counts in persons missing the G6PD enzyme. *Use caution or avoid use if you:* Have liver or kidney abnormalities; are allergic to any antimalarial medications; have abnormalities; have a G6PD deficiency; or are pregnant.
infliximab (Remicade®)	One of the new "anti-TNF" RA medications. Because of its higher cost, presently being given	3 mg/kg or 1.36 mg/lb of body weight every 8 weeks.	Over 50 percent of individuals see a benefit after the first injection, and maximum benefit	Not required.	*Possible side effects include:* Check with your doctor if you experience chills, cough, fever, skin rash, or frequent or painful urination. Allergic reactions are rare but potentially serious. The

Drug	Description	Dosage	Improvement	Side effects / Cautions	Monitoring
	to those with moderate to severe RA or those not responding to other DMMs.	(e.g., for a person weighing 64 kg, or 141 lbs, their maximum daily dose would be 416 mg.) Administered over a two-hour period intravenously (into the vein). Store in the refrigerator.	should be seen by six weeks.	risk of cancer is a potential concern. However, long-term studies are pending. The development of auto-antibodies is increased. Serious infections, multiplesclerosis–like disorder, and reduced blood counts have occurred and rarely have resulted in death. *Use caution or avoid use if you:* Are pregnant; are breast-feeding; had allergic reaction to rodents (such as rats or mice); are elderly.	
leflunomide (Arava®)	Used to treat individuals with moderate to severe RA if they do not respond to methotrexate. Can be used as a single therapy or in combination with methotrexate.	100 mg/day for three days to start then 20 mg/day thereafter as a single therapy. If taken in combination with methotrexate, 10 mg/day.	Should see improvement in one to two months.	*Possible side effects include:* Diarrhea, rash, hair loss, abnormal liver tests, lung disease, low platelets, nausea, loss of weight, severe allergy, and increased risk of infection. *Use caution or avoid use if you:* Have existing kidney or liver disease, are taking rifampin or tolbutamide. Serious liver problems, including permanent liver disease and lung disease resulting in death, have been reported.	*On starting:* AST, ALT, albumin, CBC, platelets and creatinine. *Ongoing:* AST, ALT, albumin, CBC, platelets and creatinine, monthly, or more frequently for the first six months and every eight weeks thereafter.

Generic Medication Name (Brand Name)	Use/Benefit	Average Adult Maintenance Dose Range	How Long Before It Works	Monitoring Tests	Side Effects, Cautions
leflunomide (cont'd.)					**Do not use if you are pregnant.** Because the medication remains in the blood for two years and can damage a fetus (unborn baby), the medication must be removed by a special eleven-day treatment with cholestyramine. Both women wishing to become pregnant and men (taking leflunomide) wanting to father a child must receive cholestyramine treatment.
methotrexate (Rheumatrex®)	This is most rheumatologists' therapy of choice for moderate to severe RA, as well as for mild RA not responding to one or several other DMMs. It can be taken in combination with hydroxychloroquine, sulfasalazine, gold sodium thiomalate, gold thioglucose, etanercept, infliximab.	7.5–25 mg once per week in a single dose. Taken by mouth, or by injection. If taking by mouth, take with food.	Benefits should be seen within one to two months; maximum benefit at six months.	*On starting:* CBC, creatinine, chest X-ray within the past year, hepatitis B and C serology in high-risk individuals, AST or ALT, alkaline phosphatase, albumin. *Ongoing:* CBC, platelet count, AST, albumin, and creatinine	*Possible side effects:* Decreased appetite, nausea, abdominal pain, mouth ulcers, hair loss, increased bruising, rise in liver enzyme test, or increased risk of infection. Liver damage or lung inflammation are rare but potentially serious. Toxicity is increased if there is kidney damage. *Use caution or avoid use if you:* Had or have liver damage, abuse alcohol, have viral liver disease, are obese, or have diabetes mellitus. Do not take sulfa antibiotics without speaking to your rheumatologist.

Drug	Usage	Dosage	Benefit timing	Monitoring	Possible side effects / cautions
				every four to eight weeks while on the therapy.	**Do not use if you are pregnant. As well, methotrexate must be stopped in BOTH MEN AND WOMEN three months prior to attempting to conceive a baby.**
minocycline (Minocin®)	This therapy is used in mild early RA (disease onset=two years).	200 mg per day in two doses. Taken by mouth. Take on an empty stomach.	Benefit should be seen within two to three months.	N/A	*Possible side effects:* Dizziness, vaginal infections, nausea, diarrhea, headache, skin rash with sun exposure, or increased grey skin pigmentation. Rarely, pressure in the brain or autoimmune disease such as lupus. *Use caution or avoid use if you:* Are sensitive to tetracycline medications or have sun sensitivities.
d-penicillamine (Cuprimine®) (Depen®)	Rarely used.	250 mg to 1000 mg per day in three doses. Dosage should not exceed 1000 mg. Doses higher than 750 mg per day substantially increase the chance of side effects.	Benefits should be seen in three to six months.	*On starting:* CBC, platelets, and urinalysis biweekly or when changing the dose. *Ongoing:* CBC and urinalysis monthly.	*Possible side effects:* Mouth sores; decrease in sense of taste; nausea; diarrhea; abdominal pain; itchy rash. Suppression of the ability to make blood cells (red cells, white cells, platelets) and the development of protein leakage from the kidney are rare but potentially serious. The development of other autoimmune disease are rare but can be very serious.

Generic Medication Name (Brand Name)	Use/Benefit	Average Adult Maintenance Dose Range	How Long Before It Works	Monitoring Tests	Side Effects, Cautions
d-penicillamine (cont'd.)		Taken by mouth. Take on an empty stomach.			*Use caution or avoid use if you:* Have blood or kidney disease. *Do not use if you are pregnant.* D-penicillamine can cause skin abnormalities in the fetus.
plasmapherisis (Prosorba Column®)	Used in moderate to severe RA in individuals who don't respond to multiple other DMMs.	Used weekly for twelve weeks. Can be repeated.	Benefits may not be seen until after the twelve treatments are completed.	*Before each treatment:* CBC, platelets, creatinine, albumin, electrolytes.	*Possible side effects:* Transient increases in joint swelling, joint pain and fatigue occur. Fever, chills, low blood pressure, nausea, abdominal pain, numbness and headache are common during the plasmapheresis. Inflammation of blood vessels, rash, clotting, chest pain and trouble breathing may occur. Decrease in red blood cells (hemoglobin) occurs rarely. *Use caution or avoid use:* ACE (angiotensin converting enzyme) inhibitors must be stopped at least three days before a treatment. Angiotensin-2 receptor antagonists may be used. Not to be used in

| | | | | | persons with inflammation of blood vessels or increased risk of clotting (e.g., recent heart attack or stroke). |
| Sulfasalazine (Azulfidine®) | This therapy is used in mild early RA, and in moderate to severe RA, in combination with hydroxychloroquine, sulfasalazine, and methotrexate. | 2 to 3 g per day in three to four doses. | Benefits should be seen in one to two months. | *On starting*: CBC and LFTs biweekly for the first three months.

Ongoing: CBC and LFTs every one to three months. | *Possible side effects*: Decreased appetite, nausea, vomiting, abdominal pain, and skin rash are fairly common. Suppression of the ability to make blood cells and effects on the liver are rare but potentially serious. A reversible decrease in fertility can occur in males. Can affect the blood counts in persons missing the G6PD enzyme. |

seems to work only when it is started in the first two years of RA. Oral gold (Ridura®) is used less frequently than the others, partly due to diarrhea as a side effect and partly because rheumatologists feel it is not as effective as was first thought. Hydroxychloroquine is the most commonly used. While it may be less effective than sulfasalazine, side effects are less common with hydroxychloroquine than any other DMM.

Moderate to severe RA, and Mild RA that is not responding to one, or at most two, of the above therapies. For moderate or severe RA, and for mild RA that is not responding to one, or at most two, of the above therapies, methotrexate is the current medication of choice. If a person started on hydroxychloroquine but had incomplete improvement, methotrexate might well be added to the hydroxychloroquine. Taking 1 mg/day of folic acid (a natural vitamin) reduces many of the side effects of methotrexate. Intramus-cular gold (injected by needle into the buttock) has fallen from favor in some countries but remains a highly effective medication.

If the person's RA improved with methotrexate and hydroxychloroquine but didn't experience completely controlled disease, sulfasalazine might be added to the combination. For many with RA, the "triple combination" of methotrexate, hydroxychloroquine, and sulfasalazine is very effective and safe with the appropriate monitoring. (*Caution: Sulfasalazine should not be taken by individuals allergic to sulfa.*)

Azathioprine is another medication therapy used to treat moderate to severe RA. None of the medication therapies listed above suppress the immune system—azathioprine does. It is an immunosuppresant (it acts to control RA by suppressing the body's immune system), which is why the use of this therapy is limited. Another immunosuppresant is cyclosporine. It is effective alone, and when added to methotrexate, the benefits increase. Cyclosporine has more serious side effects than azathioprine. Both azathioprine and cyclosporine are generally used in those individuals with moderate to severe RA not responding to other DMMs.

Leflunomide (Arava®) is a new immune-suppressant medication, which is about as effective as methotrexate, at least in the early studies. Leflunomide can be added to methotrexate to increase the benefit and is less expensive than the new *antitumor necrosis factor therapies* (anti-TNF).

The place of the anti-TNF therapies, etanercept (Enbrel®) and infliximab (Remicade®), in treating RA is developing as we are writing. The early studies of infliximab (always given with methotrexate) and etanercept (given alone or with methotrexate) showed dramatic therapeutic benefits. And, so far, there are no more side effects than those seen with methotrexate, and fewer lab tests are required while taking them. The most common side effects seen to date are skin reactions, where etanercept injections are given, and allergic reactions with infliximab.

Because the experience with anti-TNF therapies has not been that long, there is concern about long-term side effects, particularly cancer, infection, and other immune disease. Serious life-threatening infections have occurred. Individuals with active infections, including chronic infections such as tuberculosis (TB), should not receive anti-TNF therapies. Recently, a small number of individuals, some of whom died, have been reported to have developed multiple sclerosis-like disorders, and others exhibited marked reductions in the body's ability to make blood cells.

As with most emerging therapies, cost is an issue, and that holds true for etanercept and infliximab. In the United States, a one-year supply of either drug costs approximately $12,000. For those who are eligible for Medicare, the cost of medications given into the vein (such as infliximab) are fully covered; self-injected medications (such as etanercept) are not. Recent legislation before the U.S. Congress proposes expanded coverage to include self-injected anti-TNF therapies.

Very severe RA. For very severe systemic disease—that is, RA that affects the blood vessels and lung tissue, among other organ systems—cyclophosphamide is used. This is a powerful immunosuppressant medication that is increasingly being given intravenously (injected into a vein) in a large dose once every four weeks.

CORTICOSTEROIDS

See Table 4.4 for a list of commonly prescribed corticosteroids. Philip Hench from the Mayo Clinic won the Nobel Prize in 1950 for his discovery of corticosteroids and their powerful effect on controlling the inflammation of RA. Subsequently, the devastating side effects of prolonged high-dose therapy limited their use. The initial dramatic benefits of corticosteroids followed by the discovery of long-term costs tempered the enthusiasm of rheumatologists for all new DMMs. The benefits of corticosteroids were obvious; the side effects, less so.

Corticosteroids are now given in three ways—into joints, by mouth, and sometimes in very severe RA, by a large intravenous dose. Corticosteroids play a major, *but ideally temporary*, role in your medication therapy treatment plan. They are used primarily as a "bridge" therapy to get you through

TABLE 4.4. PRESCRIPTION CORTICOSTEROID MEDICATION THERAPIES

Generic Medication Name (Brand Name)	Use/Benefit	Average Adult Maintenance Dose Range	How Long Before It Works	Monitoring Tests	Side Effects, Cautions
corticosteroids *prednisone* (pill) (Deltasone®, Orasone®, Prednicen-M®, Sterapred®) *dexamethasone* (pill) (Decadron®, Hexadrol®) *cortisone* (pill) (Cortone Acetate®) *methylprednisolone* (joint injection) (Depo-Medrol®) *triamcinolone acetonide* (joint injection) (Kenalog®) *triamcinolone hexacetonide* (joint injection) (Aristospan®) *methylprednisolone* (intravenous) (Medrol®)	*By pill,* as a temporary therapy while waiting for DMMs to begin controlling the disease, or as long-term therapy until disease is better controlled by DMMs. *By injection,* used to treat one or two inflamed joints when otherwise the disease is well-controlled by DMMs. Taken by injection into a joint, or by pill, with food or an antacid in the morning. *By vein* (intravenous), in very severe disease.	Dosages are highly variable and depend on the individual and their disease severity and activity. **When used for periods longer than several weeks, do not stop taking abruptly. Dosage must be reduced slowly.**	By injection, benefits are seen within twenty-four to seventy-two hours. By pill, benefits are seen within twenty-four to forty-eight hours.	*Upon starting:* CBC, platelet count, creatinine, liver tests, blood sugar, and cholesterol.	*Possible side effects include:* Increased appetite, weight gain due to fat (especially over your face, upper body, and belly), fluid retention, difficulty sleeping, mood changes, heartburn, and thin skin. Corticosteroids also increase blood pressure, cholesterol, and blood sugar levels. Less commonly, they weaken the muscles, increase the chance of cataracts, elevate pressure in the eye, induce stomach ulcer, infection, permanent bone damage called osteonecrosis, nervousness or restlessness. *Use caution or avoid use if you:* Have active infection or inactive tuberculosis hypothyroidism, herpes simplex of the eye, hypertension, osteoporosis, stomach ulcer, diabetes.

the period before the DMM has a chance to work. (Remember, most DMMs can take anywhere from several weeks to six to twelve months before their full benefit is achieved.)

Corticosteroids are commonly given as an occasional injection into a severely inflamed joint—often, when the disease is well-controlled except for one or two joints, as well as early on when the disease is not controlled but several joints are particularly "bad." When this is the case, some of the injected medication "escapes" and travels to other joints in the body causing a more general benefit. This approach to corticosteroid use is highly effective in that the dose of DMM you are taking can be maintained.

Corticosteroids are also given over a period of weeks to months in pill form: usually prednisone (Deltasone®, among many other brands). Sometimes they are given in a burst—say six tablets a day, reduced to none over two to three weeks. Again, the hope is to control active inflammation while awaiting benefit from a DMM.

In very severe RA, such as when it affects the lining of the heart or lung in a major way or causes inflammation of the blood vessels, corticosteroids may be given in very large doses intravenously. This is done to gain rapid control of the disease and prevent damage. Because the drug is given in a brief burst, the side effects are usually less severe than when the same amount is given over a longer period of time.

Because corticosteroids are so effective, some individuals with RA need to remain on them for long periods of time—even years. In these cases, the lowest possible dose is used and medication to prevent osteoporosis (thin or weak bones) must be taken. The goal with corticosteroid use should be to slowly reduce the amount taken as the disease is controlled by DMMs. *It must be slowly reduced* because the corticosteroid our body's adrenal gland makes naturally in order to live is suppressed when the medication is taken in pill form, as it is in RA. Gradually tapering the dose of corticosteroid allows the body's adrenal glands to "kick in" and start making it naturally again.

If you need to incorporate long-term corticosteroid therapy into your medication plan, you should wear a "medical alert" bracelet or necklace that tells a physician you are taking prednisone all the time.

In addition to thin bones, common side effects with prolonged corticosteroid therapy include increased appetite, weight gain (especially over your face, upper body, and belly), fluid retention, difficulty sleeping, mood changes, heartburn, and thin skin. Corticosteroids also increase blood pressure, cholesterol and blood sugar levels. Less commonly, they weaken the muscles, increase the chance of cataracts, elevate pressure in the eye, and induce stomach ulcers, infection, and permanent bone damage called osteonecrosis.

The increased understanding of the complex processes that drive the immune system and cause the inflammation of RA resulted in the new anti-TNF medication therapies. A recently available therapy for individuals with severe RA who have not responded to conventional therapies is *plasmapheresis* (blood washing). Plasma is the fluid part of blood (as opposed to the cells), and plasmapheresis is the medical term for blood washing. The individual's blood is passed through a column which absorbs antibodies, including antibody complexes that are thought to be damaging, and is then returned to the body. The therapy, called the Prosorba® column, is very expensive and its exact role in the treatment of RA is only now being established.

Undoubtedly, as scientists learn more about the immune system and the inflammatory pathways involved in RA, more new therapies will be developed—and many are already at the testing stage. For example: IL-1 ra (interleukin-1 receptor antagonist) or Anakinra® is a novel therapy that is completing the final phases of clinical testing. IL-1 is a molecule that promotes the inflammation of RA. IL-1 ra limits the activity of IL-1, and diminishes the inflammation, and slows the development of erosions (bone damage) due to RA. FK-506 is a cyclosporine-like drug that is in the early phase of testing in RA.

RESEARCH INTO NEW MEDICATIONS

With only a limited number of highly effective RA medications, approved for use today, an urgent need exists to develop additional ones—medications that present fewer risks and have greater effectiveness for the person with RA. As mentioned above, several new medications are available (etanercept, infliximab, leflunomide) but more are needed.

Developing and testing new medications is a long, arduous process involving scientists of many types, physicians, pharmaceutical companies, government, and people living with the disease, to name a few. From first discovery to marketing, a medicine can take upward of ten years, and can cost hundreds of millions of dollars. The development of a new medication takes equal measures of vision, commitment, and expertise from myriad experts. However, most important, there must be a need for it. Aside from methotrexate, fewer than 20 percent of patients remain on one specific DMM for longer than three years due to lack of effectiveness, toxicity, or an increase in disease activity.

The knowledge gained from early scientific studies of a new medication form an important part of the evidence you should rely on when making decisions about trying an emerging therapy. Why? Because they help to tell the story of at least the short-term benefits and risks that a therapy may present.

CLINICAL TRIALS

The vehicle for testing an experimental medication for approval as one that can be prescribed is called a *clinical trial*. Clinical trials study new (hence experimental) medications in a group of people (known as "study participants") meeting specific criteria. Clinical trials also may test existing medications used in new ways, in new dosages, or compared to different medications. In order to receive government approval for licensing and widespread use, an experimental medication must successfully pass three phases of clinical testing, listed below.

Phase I
Determines in what dose the experimental medication is well tolerated in a small group of healthy individuals, usually twenty to eighty, and to look for possible side effects not present in laboratory tests on animals. This phase usually takes several months.

Phase II
Determines the effectiveness of the experimental medication and develop dosage guidelines in a group of individuals with the disease of interest, usually eighty to three hundred. This phase typically takes several months to two years.

Phase III
Compares the experimental medication in a large, carefully selected and closely monitored group of individuals with the disease (1,000 to 3,500) against a placebo (a dummy pill or medication that lacks the active drug) so that researchers can determine whether the experimental medication works—that is, if it is better than the placebo. Phase III trials also may compare the new medication against existing ones in order to determine its place among them. In addition, this phase monitors short-term side effects and gathers other information that will lead to the medication's safe use in the general population of individuals with the disease. This phase typically takes one to four years.

Phase IV
Phase IV studies run after an experimental medication receives government approval and are commonly referred to as "postmarketing" studies. This phase looks at the effect of the medication in a less restricted group of study

participants than were studied in Phase III. Phase IV studies are also important, because they assess the long-term benefits or side effects of a medication. This information may not have been available from earlier studies but is of great interest to people with RA and physicians alike. This phase can last anywhere from one to many years.

Clinical Trial Models

Like cars, clinical trials come in different "models." Listed below are the superior scientific models for clinical trials today.

RANDOMIZED CONTROL TRIAL (RCT)

Once accepted into the trial, the study participants are assigned randomly to a treatment therapy they will receive. Typically, there are two or three groups. One group of study participants receives the experimental medication (called the "study group"). Another may receive a placebo or "dummy medication" (called the "placebo control group"), and yet another may receive the standard medication (called the "active therapy control group").

The participants are assigned randomly so that every group will contain individuals with similar chances of responding or not responding to the new medication, the placebo, or the other active drug. Again, by comparing the response to the new medication and to the placebo allows researchers to determine if it works. By comparing the new medication response to that of other active medications, researchers learn how the new medication compares to one that is already in use.

DOUBLE-BLIND RANDOMIZED CONTROL TRIAL (RCT)

The scientific rigor of an RCT increases when *neither* the study participant *nor* the researcher knows the group assignments of the study participants (known as "blinding"). Blinding the researcher and the study participant helps to prevent influences other than the effect of the medication (called "bias") on the determination of whether the participant is improving, has a side effect, and so on. If only the participant or the researcher is unaware of which group the participant is assigned to, then the study is referred to as a "single-blind" RCT. And, while a single-blind study is less rigorous than a double-blind study, it is superior to an "un-blinded" RCT, in which both the researcher and the study participant know which group the participant is in. To prove that a medication really works, governments usually require at least two studies with random assignment, at least a placebo control group, and double-blinding. If any of these are absent, caution should be exercised in accepting that the medication being tested works—*especially if you are the one being asked to take the medication.* Uncontrolled trials are particularly of lower caliber because they have no control group to serve as a basis of comparison. In other words, the inability to compare one group to another means the study results are largely irrelevant for decision making. A strongly positive result in an uncontrolled study may well lead to calls for one or more double-blinded RCTs.

Determining the Quality or Caliber of a Clinical Trial

The following criteria determines the quality of a clinical trial.

EXPERIENCE AND REPUTATION OF THE TRIAL'S PRINCIPAL INVESTIGATOR AND THE OTHER INVESTIGATORS

The person in charge of running the trial is the "principal investigator." Make sure she or he is someone with a history of interest in clinical research, and well respected in the field of rheumatology and the research community. Check to see if the researcher has published studies in high-quality general medicine journals, such as *American Journal of Medicine, New England Journal of Medicine, Annals of Internal Medicine, British Medical Journal, Journal of the American Medication Association, Lancet,* as well as in high quality rheumatology journals such as *Arthritis and Rheumatism, British Journal of Rheumatology, Journal of Rheumatology, Annals of Rheumatic Diseases, Rheumatology, Arthritis Care and Research,* and *Seminars in Arthritis and Rheumatism.*

TYPE OF TRIAL

Is there a control group? Is the assignment to the experimental medication and the control medication(s) random? Are both the researchers *and* the study participants unaware of the treatment assignment (i.e., is it double-blind)? These are all important questions to ask when trying to determine the quality of a trial.

TRIAL OBJECTIVE AND DESIGN

A clearly defined trial objective (what is it that the new medication will improve) and the specific way that improvement will be measured largely determine what information researchers can take away from the trial. A trial that assesses whether a new medication influences a blood test may be less important to you than whether the medication improves quality of life.

TRIAL PROTOCOL

The trial protocol establishes the "rules" of the clinical trial. The protocol defines what is being studied in the clinical trial and why; the characteristics of who is allowed to participate (e.g., mild or severe disease, young or old) and how many; what tests or procedures are required before, during, and after the trial; what dosages of medication participants will take; how long the clinical trial will last; how side effects will be assessed; the participants' rights and responsibilities; and so on. A clearly described protocol makes it likely that all participants will be treated appropriately and will determine what type of person the results apply to. For instance, if people with only mild RA were included in the clinical trial, the results may not apply, or not apply to the same extent, to those with very severe disease.

The "Pros and Cons" of Participating in a Clinical Trial

As with most things in life, there are pros and cons you should consider before participating in a clinical trial.

THE PROS

- gives the study participant access to experimental therapies that may prove effective against RA: this is particularly important for individuals not responding to existing medications
- gives the study participant expert medical care and attention beyond that given by their own health care team—at no additional cost; careful monitoring for benefits and side effects during a clinical trial can often provide early detection of RA-related (or unrelated) health issues for the study participant
- gives the study participant access to experimental medications free of charge; for Phase IV clinical trials in particular, this could be a significant benefit, because newly approved therapies often can cost substantially more than older therapies when they first come on the market
- information collected during the study advances the understanding of RA treatment, thereby helping present and future generations living with the disease by giving a definitive answer

THE CONS

- your RA may not improve because of your participation
- you may experience side effects
- participating in a clinical trial can be time consuming; depending on the medication being studied and the study "protocol," you may be required to visit the clinical trial nurse or doctor much more frequently than normal to receive the medication, answer questions, or undergo tests, and you should be told how much extra time will be required
- in a single- or double-blinded randomized clinical trial, there is a chance you will not receive the experimental medication being studied; instead, you may be receiving the placebo (or dummy) medication
- depending on the question(s) the researcher is trying to answer in the trial, you may have to undergo more complex tests, such as

an endoscopy (a test in which a tube is passed through your
mouth to your stomach) in a study of ulcers from NSAIDs
- the clinical trial protocol may interfere with your lifestyle (e.g.,
you need to take the medication or visit the clinical trial site at
inconvenient times, you need to restrict your diet, etc.)

Things to Consider Before Participating

Getting high-quality results from a clinical trial relies on commitment, both
on the part of the participant and on the part of the clinical trial staff. Below
is a list of questions (along with others you may have) you should ask the
clinical trial staff before you consent (agree) to participate. (You also may
wish to ask these same questions of your rheumatologist or family doctor.)

- What is the purpose of the clinical trial? Does it sound meaning-
ful to you?
- Is there a need for the clinical trial? Are you convinced it will help
you or others with RA?
- Do I have to pay to participate? What will I pay for? Does my
insurance cover the cost(s)? What about transportation, parking,
missed meals?
- What are the potential benefits and possible side effects?
- Are the possible side effects reversible?
- How is the medication administered?
- Are there other treatment options I can try (other than the one
being studied) that may be less "risky" for me to take?
- What tests will I have to take during the course of the clinical
trial? What procedures?
- Where is the clinical trial site nearest me?
- How many visits to the clinical trial site will I have to make?
- Will I have to be in the hospital at any time during the trial? How
long?
- How long does the clinical trial last?
- What is the process for enrollment?
- If the medication I take during the clinical trial is effective, can I
still take it when the trial concludes? Will it be free and for how
long?
- What happens if the therapy does receive approval once the trial
concludes?
- If I end up on placebo, can I try the experimental therapy when
the trial concludes?
- Will I receive written results of the trial in consumer-friendly
language?
- Will my privacy be protected during and after the trial?

Remember, if you become concerned for your safety—or for any other reason—at any point during the course of the trial, you may withdraw your consent to participate. However, you are encouraged to share your concerns with the clinical trial staff before withdrawing from the study. Often, the staff can address your concerns to your satisfaction, making you comfortable to continue in the study.

Finding Out About Clinical Trials

To start with, speak to your rheumatologist about clinical trials in your area. If they are not active in arthritis research, they will likely have colleagues who are. You also can make enquiries to the rheumatology department at a university teaching hospital near you.

Both The Arthritis Foundation in the United States and The Arthritis Society in Canada fund promising new arthritis research and have information on clinical trials recruitment on their websites. The National Institutes of Health (NIH) in the United States also has in-depth information on clinical trials on its website. These and other website addresses are listed in Chapter 12.

Chapter 5

EXERCISE

"Strengthen the weak hands, and make firm the feeble knees."

—Bible, Isaiah 35:3

"Don't wait for your ship to come in. Swim out to it."

—Anonymous

Physical fitness plays a critical role in maintaining, or gaining back, optimal health—especially when living with a chronic condition like RA. The benefits of being fit touch every part of our lives—our overall energy level, sleep patterns, psychological and emotional well-being, and relationships.

Except when you are experiencing severe or sharp joint pain and noticeable swelling, exercise should be a regular part of your day. The latest research shows that physical conditioning exercise can improve your fitness level without aggravating your RA or causing a flare of symptoms.[1,2,3,4] So whether you have mild, moderate, or severe disease, exercise is an important part of your plan. However, it is important to understand that the type and intensity of exercise may need to be regulated, depending on your disease activity.

Getting started with an exercise program and making it part of your daily routine can be challenging, even a little intimidating, at first. But fear not—you can do it. By starting slowly and learning proper exercise techniques from qualified health care professionals, you will be well on your way toward having a body optimally equipped to deal with the physical challenges RA presents.

EXERCISE IS A GOOD THING

If ever a disease tried to trick, cajole, and force a body to stop moving, RA is it. With hot, swollen joints and the fatigue that often accompanies RA, it can be a true struggle—sometimes even impossible—to maintain your previous level of physical activity. But whether a few or nearly all of the body's joints are affected, you must do everything in your power to keep your joints mobile.

Where rheumatologists once prescribed bed rest for people with RA, they now recommend range-of-motion, strengthening, and aerobic exercise—all with good reason. Incorporating exercise into your daily routine can help control pain, inflammation and stiffness, help you get a better night's sleep and awake refreshed, and improve your self-esteem and sense of well-being.[5]

And like your medication plan, your exercise plan should be designed to address your specific needs, taking into account your diagnosis, the level of your disease activity, previous and present functioning, lifestyle, and exercise goals.

GETTING STARTED

Whether you've been active in the past, or are starting an exercise program for the first time, start out slowly. Talk to your rheumatologist about your decision to include exercise as part of your treatment plan. Ask if they have any specific concerns or suggestions that you should be aware of before starting. Likely, they will caution you about doing too much, too soon, and, wisely, refer you to a registered physiotherapist—*but make sure it is one who has experience designing exercise programs for people with RA.*

The physiotherapist is an important part of your health care team when it comes to exercise. At your first visit, expect to spend the majority of the appointment time answering questions to ascertain your past and present fitness level, and having a thorough physical examination done to assess how RA is affecting your joints. Make sure you take along a pair of loose fitting shorts and a T-shirt to wear on this first and subsequent visits. The physiotherapist needs to be able to see your knees, ankles, elbows, shoulders, and so on, to check for visible swelling and heat in the joints before making recommendations for your exercise plan. For more information about physiotherapy, see Chapter 3.

GO FOR THE GOAL

Whenever we pursue a long-term goal, such as changing careers, purchasing a house or car, or planning a dream vacation, we identify steps to take in order to reach the goal. The same is true for your exercise program. Whether your long-term goal is to maintain your ability to perform daily activities, walk through Central Park, swim with dolphins, or hike in the Rocky Mountains, setting goals will help to get you there.

In consultation with your physiotherapist, identify the steps you need to take to accomplish your long-term goal. Start with the smaller, more easily achievable steps first: Feeling a sense of accomplishment early on is a terrific exercise motivator and will help you keep your eye on your long-term goal.

Another way to keep your goal in sight is to write it down on paper and post it on your home office door, bathroom mirror, or anywhere you will see it on a daily basis. Consider it your exercise contract with yourself. Make sure that as time passes, you record your progress as well as make note of any problems you encounter along the way in your health journal. Share your successes with your health care team on a regular basis, and ask them for solutions to problems if you're having difficulty finding them on your own. Remember, they are some of your biggest supporters and will be happy to help.

Finally, remember to exercise at your own pace and mix up your routine every month or so. For example, reverse the order in which you perform the exercises; if you usually start with lower body exercises, change the routine and start with the upper body for several weeks. As well, visit your physiotherapist every three or four months to learn new or modified exercises to add to your routine—keeping the exercise routine "fresh" will help you stay interested in it and keep it fun.

BEFORE, DURING, AND AFTER EXERCISE

With any exercise plan, there are some guidelines you should know about—and follow—in order to meet with success. These guidelines apply to Olympic-caliber athletes and individuals with RA alike. *As a precaution, do not attempt the exercises described in this chapter without first checking with your rheumatologist or physiotherapist.*

Before

- To get your body ready to exercise, apply heat or cold to the joints most affected by the disease.
- Choose cold if you are experiencing pain and swelling or warmth in the joint. If you don't have a "gel pack," ice in a Zip Lock freezer bag or a package of frozen vegetables, wrapped in a thin towel, will do the trick. Apply cold no longer than ten to fifteen minutes.
- If the joint has pain but no warmth or swelling, then consider heat as an alternative to cold. The best source of moist heat for the total body is a warm whirlpool bath or shower. To warm specific areas, apply a hot water bottle, heating pad, or hot moist towel for approximately fifteen to twenty minutes. Use mild to moderate heat only—it is not a case of the hotter the better.
- Always wear appropriate clothing (for example, too long or baggy pants can get in the way), shoes, and any shoe orthotics or joint splints that may have been prescribed for you when exercising.

Also, be sure to use exercise equipment properly; using it improperly can cause as much harm as it can good.

- To prevent injury and prepare your body for strengthening and cardiovascular exercise, take each of your joints through its complete range of motion, particularly those to be used during the exercise session.

During

- Performing each exercise with the proper technique is essential to preventing injury and to producing the best results. Whether standing, sitting, or lying down, try exercising in front of a mirror to ensure that you are executing the exercises as your physiotherapist showed them to you.
- Be very deliberate in your movements for each exercise. Do each repetition as though you were being filmed in "slow motion." Don't worry if you cannot get through all of the repetitions: Doing each exercise correctly is more important. As you gain strength, you can add more until you reach your target number of repetitions.
- Make sure your body has the oxygen it needs to exercise effectively and efficiently—breath. *Take one breath out on exertion and one slow breath in as you relax.*
- During exercise, you will likely notice an increase in your heartbeat and your muscles will begin to fatigue during the exercise session: These are normal bodily functions and should not cause you alarm.

After

- After exercising, "cool down" gradually for approximately ten minutes. The cool down phase allows your heart to return to its normal resting rate and helps to keep your muscles from tightening up and being sore afterwards.
- The cool down comprises gentle stretches for the muscles and joints used during the exercise routine. Your physiotherapist should show you stretches that are appropriate for each type of exercise in your routine. Do each stretch slowly and hold for twenty to thirty seconds. Avoid bouncing movements, and don't overstretch around unstable joints or where you are experiencing pain.

EXERCISE WARNING SIGNS

Protecting and preventing joint damage during exercise is critical in RA. If you experience increased joint pain, warmth, or swelling because of exercise, see your rheumatologist or physiotherapist to discuss ways to modify the exercise or exercises causing the problem.

As well, be aware of your body's signals. If you experience pain or cramping in a muscle, stop and gently stretch it until the pain stops. Continue the exercise slowly. If you become dizzy during exercise, stop the exercise and sit down. Two common causes for dizziness during exercise include not eating beforehand and not drinking enough water during exercise. If the dizziness is severe, if you notice your chest getting "tight," or if you become severely short of breath, stop exercising immediately and contact your family physician.

EXERCISE TO GET AND KEEP YOU MOBILE

The first type of exercise your physiotherapist will want you to incorporate into your daily routine is range of motion exercise, or "ROM." ROM exercise focuses on a specific joint and moves it through its entire normal range of motion in each possible direction. The primary joints requiring ROM exercise are: fingers and hands, wrists, elbows, shoulders, hips, knees, ankles, and toes.

The key benefits of ROM exercise are:

- maintains or increases joint flexibility
- reduces stiffness and pain
- helps you to perform daily activities

ROM exercise should be done at least once, but preferably twice each day, morning and evening. Morning ROM exercises are best performed after you shower; the warm water will help loosen the joints before you begin. Taking your joints through another set of ROM exercise in the evening will help significantly with morning stiffness.[6]

Each joint should be moved through its full ROM for three to ten repetitions, also called "reps," once or twice each day. Your entire ROM routine will take approximately ten to fifteen minutes. Have your physiotherapist demonstrate each of the exercises first so that you can watch and ask questions, and then perform the exercise yourself with the physiotherapist watching and critiquing. Take along a family member or friend for "training" if you think you may need help remembering all of the exercises you are shown, and in case you may need their help to exercise down the road. You should have at least two to four instructional ROM exercise sessions with your physiotherapist before starting the program at home.

If you have joints that are very hot and swollen, gently move your joint through one full ROM. Doing just one repetition will help keep the joint mobile during periods of increased inflammation. If you're having difficulty moving the joint on your own, ask for help from your "trained" family member or friend.

ROM exercise is a cornerstone of rehabilitation after joint injury or surgery, but usually requires the assistance of a physiotherapist—especially the first few weeks after the surgery.

One last bit of advice on ROM exercise: Daily activities such as gardening, house cleaning, grocery shopping, and so on do not count as ROM exercise. These activities do not work the joints through their entire range of motion, and should not replace ROM exercise in your plan.

Below are a few of the ROM exercises your physiotherapist may show you. Many can be performed both standing and sitting. (Exercise illustrations and their descriptive text used with permission by The Arthritis Society of Canada, BC and Yukon Division.)

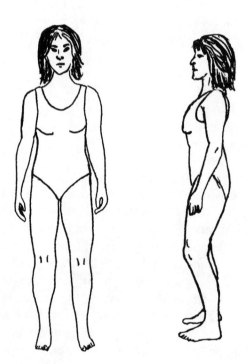

Fig. 5.1. **Basic Standing Starting Position**.
For standing ROM exercises, assume the above position at the start of each illustrated exercise. Keep your back straight, abdominals pulled up and in, shoulders back but relaxed, head centered on neck, chin in, knee joints unlocked and feet shoulder-width apart.

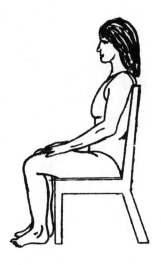

Fig. 5.2. **Basic Seated Starting Position**.
For seated ROM exercises, keep the back straight and firmly against the back of the chair, abdominals pulled up and in, shoulders back but relaxed, head centered on neck, chin in, knees bent and feet flat on the floor shoulder width apart and hands resting lightly on the thighs.

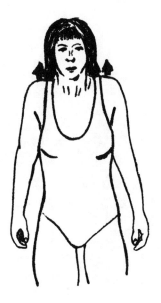

Fig. 5.3. **Shoulder Shrugs**.
Raise both shoulders up toward the ears, hold three seconds. Relax. Concentrate on completely relaxing the shoulders as they come down. Do not tilt the head or body in either direction and do not hunch shoulders forward or pinch shoulder blades together. Can be performed standing or sitting.

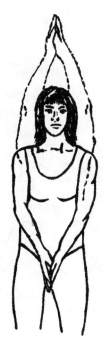

Fig. 5.4. Forward Arm Reach.
Put hands together. Raise hands up and over head as high as possible, keeping the elbows straight.

Variation:
Do one arm at a time or use one arm to assist the other if necessary.

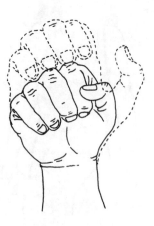

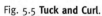

Fig. 5.5 Tuck and Curl.
With hand open and fingers straight, bend the tips of your fingers to touch the base of your fingers (like a cat's clawing motion). Then curl fingers into your palm, making a loose fist. Straighten fingers and repeat.

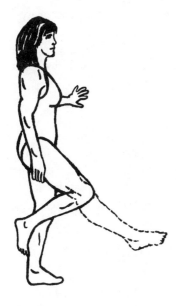

Fig. 5.6. **Knee Bends**.
Stand with back or left side against a wall.
Bend right knee bringing thigh to ninety
degrees. Straighten right knee; then bend
it again. Lower right leg with bent knee.
Ankles and toes are relaxed. Repeat with
left.

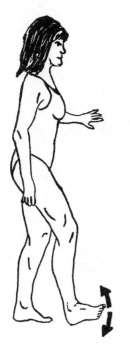

Fig. 5.7. **Ankle Bends**.
Stand with back against wall, or holding
onto the back of a chair, weight on left foot
and right knee slightly bent. Pull right foot
up, then down. Repeat with left foot. Keep
toes relaxed if you are prone to foot muscle
cramping.

EXERCISE TO GET AND KEEP YOU STRONG

The second type of exercise your physiotherapist will discuss with you is *strengthening exercise*—exercise designed to maintain or improve muscle strength that provides support for your joints.

There are two types of strengthening exercise: isometric and isotonic. Both can help you to improve your muscle strength, endurance, and mobility *without making your RA worse.*

Isometric exercise

Isometric exercise is the contraction or "tightening" of a specific muscle *without joint movement.* Because you use your own body to provide the resistance, these require no special equipment and can be done anywhere, any time. Isometric exercise is especially useful when you first develop RA, and for times during the course of your disease when one or several of your joints are more painful and swollen than normal.

Key benefits of isometric exercise are:

- maintains muscle size
- improves muscle tone
- develops muscle strength required for strenuous, weight-bearing activities
- develops muscle strength to prepare for joint surgery or replacement

To get the most out of isometric exercise, you should be doing it every day. Do five to ten reps for each muscle contraction exercise, holding each contraction for six seconds—*but no more than six seconds.*

Because this type of exercise restricts blood flow through the muscle being contracted, it can increase muscle soreness after exercise. Isometric exercise also increases the blood flow in the areas around the muscle, which (rarely) can result in an increase in blood pressure.

Fig. 5.8 is an example of an isometric exercise.

Isotonic exercise

Isotonic exercise focuses on muscle resistance *and* joint movement performed at a faster pace. Muscle resistance comes in the form of your own body weight, added weight, or exercise equipment offering resistance. Like ROM exercise, many isotonic exercises can be performed on your own at home.

Key benefits of isotonic exercise are:

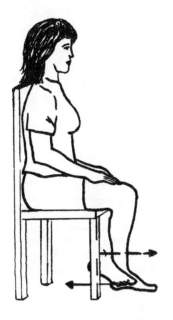

Fig. 5.8. Isometric Leg Exercise.
Sitting in a straight-backed chair with crossed ankles and knees bent, push forward with your back leg while pressing backward with your front leg. Press evenly with both legs for six seconds, making sure that neither one moves during exertion.

- maintains or increases muscle strength against resistance
- increases endurance
- improves blood flow through joint tissue
- promotes strong bones and cartilage
- improves ability to take part in daily and recreational activities

To get the most out of your isotonic exercise plan, do the exercises two to three times weekly on alternate days. Start by performing eight to ten reps for each exercise, using just your own body weight for resistance. When you can complete eight to ten reps comfortably over three to four weeks, add a one- to two-pound resistance or weights to your body or the equipment. If you are unable to move the joint with weight through its outer limits of range of motion, go as far as you can before you experience pain.

Because isotonic exercise involves joint movement and bearing of weight, take care to protect the joint during exercise. Remember, RA inflammation weakens the muscles around the joint, causing it to be less stable: ensure that you are using proper exercise technique to avoid unnecessary stress to joints. In addition, use splints (like wrist and knee support devices) to support and properly align joints during weight-bearing exercise. (In general, try to avoid bearing, picking up, or holding weight with involved hands and wrists.) If at any time you should experience severe joint pain during exercise, stop immediately.

Fig. 5.9 is an example of an isotonic exercise.

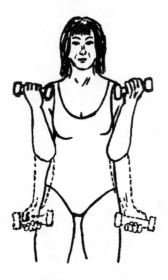

Fig. 5.9. Isometric Arm Exercise.
Standing or sitting, holding a light weight in each hand with arms relaxed by the sides, slowly bend one elbow, bringing the weight toward the shoulder, then releasing it slowly down again. Repeat with the other arm.

Range-of-Motion, Isometric, and Isotonic Exercise in Water

ROM, isometric, and isotonic exercise done in water—preferably warm water (approximately 85° F)—is particularly RA-friendly. The majority of your body weight is lifted from primary weight-bearing joints such as your feet, ankles, knees, and hips, allowing for freer and less painful movement. Water-based workouts have an excellent safety record because the water offers both support to joints and resistance to muscles.

As in land-based exercise, your water workouts should include both a warmup and cool down routine. Begin and end each session with some ROM exercises. Do three to eight reps of each ROM exercise, and remember to move through the joint's motion *fully and slowly*. (Moving your body part too fast through the water creates resistance and makes it isotonic rather than ROM exercise.)

Once you are warm and your joints are feeling relaxed and relatively free of pain, do eight to ten reps of each prescribed isotonic exercise two to three times weekly. After three to four weeks of well-tolerated exercise, add one- to two-pound weights (designed for use in the water) to increase the resistance and improve on your endurance.

Exercise and hot tubs

Soaking for ten or fifteen minutes in a hot tub set at a temperature of 95 to 104°F can be an excellent way to prepare for, and end, exercise sessions. It can warm up muscles, decrease joint pain and stiffness, and ease movement of joints.

However, use of a hot tub is not for everyone. If you have active inflammation and heat in your joints, have a preexisting lung or heart condition, low or high blood pressure, diabetes, multiple sclerosis, skin irritation or other serious illness, check with your rheumatologist before using a hot tub. If you are pregnant, do not use a hot tub or sauna. If at any time while using a hot tub you feel weak, dizzy, or nauseous, get out of the water immediately—ask for help if necessary.

EXERCISE TO GET AND KEEP YOU FIT

The third type of exercise in your PLAN TO WIN is aerobic or cardiovascular exercise. Aerobic exercise strengthens the heart and lungs by using large muscle groups (e.g., quadriceps and hamstrings): Walking, bicycling, and swimming are good examples of aerobic exercise.

Key benefits of aerobic exercise are:

- improves heart and lung function
- helps control weight
- improves strength
- reduces inflammation
- reduces joint pain
- improves self-esteem and self-confidence

To benefit from aerobic exercise, you should do some form of it for twenty to thirty continuous minutes three (to maintain fitness level) to four (to improve fitness level) times weekly. If you haven't been doing aerobic exercise on a regular basis, you may need to work your way up to thirty minutes of exercise. Start by doing five to ten minutes walking a couple of times each day, with the goal of working towards twenty to thirty minutes exercise in one daily session.

Here's what your aerobic exercise plan might look like:

- Monday   Brisk walk in the park
- Wednesday   Riding a stationary or regular bicycle
- Friday   Water-based aerobic class or swimming
- Saturday   Walk/bike cross-training (ten minutes
                    treadmill walking, ten minutes stationary
                    bike riding).

To maximize the benefit of your aerobic workout, your heart should beat between 60 to 70 percent of its age-predicted maximal heart rate per minute. To determine your age predicted maximal heart rate per minute, subtract your age in years from 220, and multiply that figure by 60 to 75

TABLE 5.1.

Age	Beats per Minute Range
20	120–150
25	117–146
30	114–142
35	111–139
40	108–135
45	105–131
50	102–127
55	99–124
60	96–120
65	93–116
70	90-112
75	87–109
80	84–105
85+	81–101

percent. For example, here is the calculation for the average forty-five-year-old person working at 70 percent of their age predicted maximal heart rate per minute:

220 - 45 = 175 x 70% = 122 beats per minute.

This calculation provides you with a conservative estimate of your maximal heart rate per minute range. Be sure to take your heart rate during and after aerobic exercise to ensure that you are working within your recommended range. (See Table 5.1.)

Depending on your fitness level, and in consultation with your GP, rheumatologist or fitness consultant, you may be able to exercise at higher levels. *However, just like with ROM, isometric, and isotonic exercise, talk to your GP, physiotherapist, or fitness consultant to agree on what your maximal heart rate per minute should be before beginning an aerobic exercise program.*

EXERCISING YOUR OPTIONS

When your RA is well controlled by your exercise and treatment plan and you want to expand your exercise horizon, think about including recreational and athletic activities you may have enjoyed before developing the disease—or even ones you've never tried before.

To start with, every effort should be made to prepare your mind and body for recreational and athletic exercise. Discuss your desire to pursue more physically intense activities with your rheumatologist and physiotherapist. Explain to them that trying to incorporate these types of exercise into your life is important to you. Ask for their professional advice on RA-friendly sports and/or recreational activities.

Depending on your disease activity, strength, and athletic ability, snow skiing, jogging, rollerblading, mountain biking, or tennis may be options to try out. While these types of activities are fun and help to restore a part of yourself you may have "lost" when RA arrived on your doorstep, be aware that they do pose some risks to your health. Let's use rollerblading as an example. You should start by making a list of the "pros and cons" of learning to rollerblade:

Pros
- I would be able to join along with my friends.
- It would help to vary my aerobic exercise routine.
- It would help me to feel like a "normal" person.
- Apart from the cost of rental or purchase of equipment, it's an affordable activity.

Cons
- There is a possibility that I might fall and injure myself.
- I might feel pressured to keep up with my friends.
- I might get overly tired from the activity.

Once the list is made, you have a good idea why you want to learn to rollerblade, and you know what concerns you have about learning. Look at each one of the "cons" as if it were a problem and see if you can find a solution. For example, possible solutions for the second and third "cons" listed are:

- rollerblade with friends who are "beginners" too
- share your concern with one of your friends, and ask if they would be willing to go a bit slower to give you some pointers or to keep you company
- pace yourself; go out for ten or fifteen minutes at a time to begin with, and as you become a better and stronger rollerblader, go out for longer periods

Finding a solution to the first "con" (the possibility of falling and injuring yourself) may not be entirely possible. Many people learning to rollerblade—whether or not they have RA—fall, and sometimes end up hurting themselves. Knowing that, ask yourself if you still want to learn to rollerblade. If the answer is yes, do whatever it takes to minimize your risk of falling and sustaining an injury:

- rent or purchase quality equipment, including protective braces and padding for your knees, wrists, hands, elbows, and head
- wear all of the protective braces and padding each time you go out, even after you get the hang of it

- wear long pants and long-sleeved shirts
- go slowly; learn at a pace that's comfortable for you, regardless of the skill level of those you rollerblade with

If you decide against rollerblading after all, look for another exercise option, one where the pros outweigh the cons.

One last reminder about joint and muscle safety before and after recreational and athletic exercise: Apply ice or heat according to the guidelines given in the *Before, During, and After Exercise* section of this chapter. Make sure to take your joints through their full range of motion before starting the activity, and gently stretch the muscles worked afterward. If you experience increased pain or swelling longer than two hours after exercise, do less the next time. This will allow you to safely and gradually develop more strength and stamina.

Chapter 6

DIET, NUTRITION, AND COMPLEMENTARY AND ALTERNATIVE MEDICINE

"Good health and good sense are two of life's greatest blessings."

—*Publius Syrus*

Your PLAN TO WIN would not be complete without considering the role of diet and nutrition. A healthy diet will help you maintain ideal body weight and prevent undue stress on weight-bearing joints; provide your body with adequate energy stores; help support your immune system to fight common illnesses such as colds and flu; and maintain adequate levels of nutrients in your body.

There is unanimity among rheumatologists, GPs, and registered dieticians/ nutritionists that a nutritionally sound diet delivers health benefits for people with RA. Much is known about the relationship between RA and diet, but few health care practitioners treating the disease pay attention to this area.

RA is a chronic health condition for which western medicine's most powerful medications fail to bring a cure. For the moderate to severe disease category (which describes the majority of RA cases), even control of the disease is a major battle. Not surprisingly, people with RA can be especially vulnerable to false claims of cure—claims that can be costly in terms of money and even more costly in terms of proven treatment delayed.

Over the years, hundreds of newspaper and magazine articles and books have reported on "dietary treatments" or "cures" for arthritis: elimination diets, shark cartilage, chicken collagen, vitamin C, New Zealand green-lipped mussel extract, glucosamine sulfate, and the list goes on. All claim to control or cure the disease; most bring no symptom relief for people with RA. Not one is scientifically *proven* to work against RA.

It is normal and natural to fear the side effects of western medication, and possibly have a preference for using "natural" remedies. However, be aware that natural does not necessarily mean harmless, and a decision to try such remedies should never mean that you abandon or delay conventional medication therapy—to do so would be playing "Russian roulette" with your joints (see Chapter 4).

To avoid falling prey to the expense and false hope of unproven claims, make this commitment to yourself as the leader of your healthcare team: Whatever dietary or natural plan you read, hear about, or have recommended to you (by a healthcare practitioner or anyone else), ask to see the research which supports its claim. Before making a decision, look at the numbers and weigh the known benefits and potential risks, just as you would if you were making any other major life decision, such as buying a car or a home.

Hundreds, if not thousands, of dietary and herbal therapies are lauded as effective treatments or cures for arthritis, but few are proven. This chapter discusses a specific few for which evidence of a benefit does exist. However, it is an overview only. If you wish to learn more about diet, nutrition, and complementary and alternative medicine in RA, go to a trusted source. Talk to your rheumatologist, GP, or a registered dietician, or see The Arthritis Foundation's excellent book, *The Arthritis Foundation's Guide to Alternative Therapies*, by Judith Horstman. (See Chapter 12.)

THE ROLE OF DIET AND NUTRITION IN RA

How much food you eat and the type of food you eat have an important effect on how well you live with RA. Because the physical symptoms of pain and inflammation make shopping, preparing, *sometimes even eating*, challenging, many people with RA have diets that include many pre-packaged or fast foods high in saturated fat. Eating too much or too many of the wrong foods often results in weight gain, as well as inadequate intake of vitamins and minerals. Adding excess weight to your skeletal (skeleton) system while it is already dealing with RA inflammation puts additional stress on your weight-bearing joints (the hips, knees, and ankles).

On the opposite end of the weight spectrum is being *underweight*. One study that looked at the nutritional status of individuals with RA showed that 26 percent were actually malnourished.[1] One explanation for malnourishment unrelated to the quantity of food being eaten is RA's effect on the metabolism. Fever, a common component when inflammation is present, increases the caloric requirements to maintain body weight.[2] Your appetite may be suppressed by the symptoms of pain and fatigue or by chemicals produced by the RA inflammation process itself. As well, the nature of RA and some of the medications make it challenging for the body to maintain adequate levels of certain nutrients, and reduces the body's ability to fight off infection and to heal quickly, resulting in low body weight.

TABLE 6.1

Food Group	Recommended Number of Servings per Day
Bread, Cereal, Rice and Pasta	6 to 11
Vegetable	3 to 5
Fruit	2 to 4
Milk, Yogurt, and Cheese	2 to 3
Meat (preferably lean or low fat)	2 to 3
	(5 oz to 7 oz total)

One way to motivate yourself to eat healthfully is to think of food as "fuel" (calories). The right kind of fuel, and proper amounts of it, can give you more energy to maintain activities of daily living, help you reach or maintain your ideal weight, and reduce your risk of other illnesses or disease. Eating from all five food groups (see Table 6.1) every day will, in part, ensure that your body has the right fuel to make new cells, grow tissue and bone, and maintain a balanced nutritional state.

A balanced diet is made up of three kinds of fuel: carbohydrates, protein, and fat. Eating the right amount of each is key to achieving good nutritional health: Ideally, 30 percent of your daily caloric intake comes from protein, 40 percent from carbohydrates, and 30 percent from fat. However, even though most people have the best intentions of eating a well-balanced diet, they sometimes fall short on nutrient intake. Many people take vitamin and mineral supplements to make up for the shortfall. These can offer benefits that are both safe and effective, when taken in consultation with a health professional.

Supplements may help when:

- your hectic lifestyle frequently keeps you from eating the recommended number of servings of each category in the food guide pyramid (available from your local public health office)
- you are on a very low calorie weight loss diet
- you are elderly and not eating as much as you should
- you are a strict vegetarian
- you cannot drink milk or eat cheese and yogurt
- you are a woman of childbearing age who does not get enough folate from fruits, vegetables, beans, and grains

If any one or several items from the list above apply to you, you might consider contacting a registered dietitian for help in evaluating your eating patterns and determining whether—and which—nutritional supplements are right for you.

NUTRITIONAL FITNESS

By incorporating a healthy diet into your plan to win, you stand the best chance of maintaining the forty-eight nutrients the body needs to function at optimum level day to day. Nevertheless, because RA and some of the medications affect the body's nutritional state, you may need to incorporate supplements as well. Knowing why you need them, which ones you need, and how they may interact with your RA medications is important. Some supplements are toxic in excessive quantities, and many interact negatively with RA and other medications you may be taking. Again, contacting a registered dietician will ensure that you are using dietary supplements in the safest way possible, and be sure to discuss supplements with your rheumatologist as well.

Calcium and Vitamin D

Calcium (a mineral) and vitamin D (a fat soluble vitamin) are two key nutrients that work to keep the body's bones healthy and strong. People with RA need to take extra care to ensure their diet includes adequate amounts of both. Simply from having the disease they are at risk of developing osteoporosis (losing bone strength or density). This is because the molecules that cause RA inflammation weaken the bones, and this process, combined with decreased physical activity experienced by many people with RA, increases the likelihood of bone thinning and subsequent fracture.

You also may be at risk for having decreased calcium and vitamin D levels in your body if you:

- have a previous diagnosis of osteoporosis
- take corticosteroid medications such as prednisone
- are female
- have a family history of osteoporosis
- have inadequate amounts of physical activity or exercise
- have had RA for a length of time
- are disabled
- have a low body mass (slight of build)
- smoke cigarettes
- consume excessive amounts of alcohol

If any one of these factors affects you, it's important to monitor your daily calcium and vitamin D intake closely to ensure that you are getting adequate amounts of each one. To prevent osteoporosis, the average adult needs to consume 1,000 to 1,500 milligrams (mg) of calcium and 400 to 800 International Units (IU) of vitamin D each day. However, be careful not to exceed your daily requirement of vitamin D, as too much can actually lead to bone thinning.

Table 6.2

Food	Amount	Calcium Content
Milk, 2%	1 cup (250 ml)	315 mg
Yogurt	4 oz (125 g)	176 mg
Swiss Cheese	1 ½ oz (45 g)	432 mg
Cheddar Cheese	1 ½ oz (45 g)	324 mg
Broccoli	1 stalk	158 mg
Sardines (canned with bones)	7 each, medium	393 mg
Salmon (canned, with bones)	3 oz (90 g)	100 mg
Almonds	½ cup (125 ml)	175 mg
Rhubarb, cooked	½ cup (125 ml)	112 mg

By helping the body to absorb calcium, vitamin D plays an essential role in maintaining skeletal health. For the individual not challenged with RA, simply going outside and enjoying the sunshine, which stimulates the production of this nutrient, and eating small amounts of food rich in vitamin D, are enough to ensure the body is getting sufficient amounts. For the individual whose nutritional balance is compromised by RA, adequate amounts of time outdoors may not be enough to ensure appropriate intake. As such, you will want to assess how much vitamin D your typical daily diet includes, and ensure the vitamin supplement you take gives you enough extra to meet your body's daily requirements.

Taking calcium and vitamin D supplements with a light meal will enhance absorption; however, be aware that certain foods can actually interfere with absorption. Foods high in phosphate (like carbonated beverages), animal protein, caffeine, soybeans, and cocoa can work against the body's ability to absorb calcium. As well, avoid taking iron with calcium; the effectiveness of both is reduced when you do so. See Table 6.2 for good food sources of calcium.

For women whose diets do not provide adequate amounts of calcium and vitamin D, a dietary supplement is required. Calcium comes in a variety of forms, but the one with the highest actual calcium content, least expensive, and most easily absorbed is calcium carbonate.

Women with RA are at greater risk of osteoporosis than men because they have less bone to begin with. At the menopause, women start to lose bone strength very rapidly and often, action must be taken. When you reach the menopause, you should discuss the merits of estrogen therapy with your rheumatologist, gynecologist, or family doctor.

Corticosteroids, such as prednisone, can result in osteoporosis. It is now recommended that women or men receiving prednisone 7.5 mg per day or for more than three months also take medication to prevent osteoporosis. A number of medications have been shown to work.

In the past, osteoporosis could only be detected on X-ray. But by the time osteoporosis became apparent on X-ray, the individual may have already lost half of their bone strength. Fortunately, bone strength can now be accurately measured with bone density testing machines. Women with RA should have bone density measured within several years of developing RA, if they need corticosteroids such as prednisone (7.5 mg per day for more than 3 months), and at menopause.

Omega-3 and Omega-6 Fatty Acids

Numerous scientific studies have reported on the positive health benefits of omega-3 type fatty acids (eicosapentaenoic [EPA] and docosahexaenoic [DHA]). These reports show that a diet with adequate amounts of this type of fat helps prevent heart disease and some forms of cancer, and most important to you, suppresses inflammation, the key symptom of RA. Two studies in particular looked at people with *mild, stable RA* taking a fish oil supplement—an excellent source of omega-3 fatty acids—and those taking a placebo ("dummy" pill). Those taking the supplement experienced reduced inflammation and were actually able to decrease the amount of nonsteroidal anti-inflammatory drugs (NSAID) they were taking.[3] Some experienced fewer tender joints and were able to stop their NSAID completely.[4]

Not all rheumatologists are ready to hop on the omega-3 fatty acid bandwagon, but there is enough evidence to support the claim that it helps in part to control RA inflammation. So what does that mean for you? In addition to making sure your diet contains enough calcium and vitamin D, you will want to ensure that the lion's share of your dietary fat comes from omega-3 fatty acids. That means eating a minimum of two to three meals per week of coldwater fish (salmon, trout, anchovy, among others) and cooking with olive or flaxseed oils.

Another fatty acid thought to be effective at reducing inflammation is gamma-linolenic acid (GLA) or omega-6. Prime sources of GLA are evening primrose and borage plants. Not many foods contain GLA in large quantities, so if you wish to take it, you will need to take it in pill form. Again, speak to a registered dietician to determine whether you need a supplement, and, if so, how much you should take and what source of GLA is best.

The Vegetarian Diet and RA

Whether a vegetarian diet benefits the person with RA has not been proved. In other words, not enough randomized clinical trials on large numbers of people with RA over long periods of time have been conducted. Having said that, there are numerous *general* health benefits delivered by a vegetarian diet. One that includes milk products and eggs (called "lacto-ovo-vegetarian") and a variety of fruits, vegetables, and grains can be low in animal fat, high in antioxidants and vitamins and high in fiber.[5]

To get adequate amounts of vitamins and nutrients from a lacto-ovo-vegetarian diet, daily intake should include:

- six to eleven servings of grain products
- three to five servings of vegetables
- two to four servings of fruit
- two to three servings of milk
- two to three servings of beans (legumes)
- sparingly of fat and sugars

For those who choose a strict vegetarian diet (called "vegan") that only includes plant-based foods, supplements with adequate amounts of vitamin B12 (derived from animal products), vitamin D, and calcium (derived from milk and bony fish, among others) are required.

UNPROVEN DIETS

Elimination Diets and Fasting

There has long been public belief that some forms of arthritis are caused by certain foods, or additives used to enhance flavor or preserve foods. However, in RA, there is scant scientific evidence to support such a belief. While some people with RA may react to certain foods in a way that causes their symptoms to worsen, there is no one food or group of foods that has been shown to cause the disease or make it worse. In other words, for every person with RA whose symptoms worsen after eating a specific food—say, tomatoes—there is a multitude for whom tomatoes pose no negative effect.

As for fasting, one study of short-term fasting in people with RA showed some benefit,[6] and another showed the effect only lasted as long as the study participants did not eat.[7] Whether the benefit occurred because specific foods were eliminated during the fast, or whether they benefited from a suppressed immune system due to the reduction in calorie intake, is unclear. However, one thing is certain: Fasting is not a long-term solution to RA.

So where do fasting and elimination diets fit into the PLAN TO WIN? If you believe there is a certain food, or food group, which makes you feel worse after eating it, with the help of a registered dietician, try eliminating it from your daily diet for a period of time and use your health journal to record how you feel. Elimination diets typically start with a one-to-two-day fasting period (water and fruit juices only) to purge the body of all food, and usually last for months. During this time, foods are introduced one at a time to determine whether the person has a reaction to them: In RA, a relevant reaction would be one or a combination of increased joint swelling, pain, or stiffness.

When following a restricted diet, record your intake, and ask yourself on a weekly basis if your joints are less swollen and painful? If you consistently answer "no" to this question throughout the duration of the diet, it is certain that diet does not cause or relieve your RA symptoms.

Again, elimination and fasting diets should never be tried unless in consultation with your rheumatologist and a registered dietician.

COMPLIMENTARY AND ALTERNATIVE MEDICINE (CAM)

Visit any health food store or pharmacy today and you'll find the shelves loaded with myriad remedies and books promising to "cure" or "naturally" treat arthritis. And, of course, numerous alternative health practitioners offer healing services privately, such as naturopaths, homeopaths, and practitioners of traditional Chinese Medicine.

Medical researchers define CAM as any intervention (treatment approach) not taught widely in medical schools nor generally available in U.S. hospitals.[8] In the complementary and alternative medicine community, CAM is defined in a slightly different way: "Alternative medicine describes independent healing systems outside the realm of western medical theory and practice or mainstream medicine. Complementary medicine describes therapies that are used along with mainstream medicine."[9]

In general, CAM includes traditional Chinese medicine (TCM), diet therapies, nutritional and herbal supplementation, naturopathy, massage, chiropractic, and Ayurveda, among others. A national survey conducted in the United States in 1997 reported that Americans spent an estimated $27 billion on alternative medicine that year.[10] In Canada, the amount was about $3.8 billion.[11]

CAM enjoys wild popularity in other countries, too. In a twelve-month period, substantial percentages of the populations of Denmark (10 percent),[12] Finland (33 percent)[13], and Australia (49 percent)[14] used at least one form of CAM.

So it seems that more and more people around the world have turned to CAM, especially those with chronic conditions like RA. It is not difficult to understand why: Many people appreciate the experience of visiting a CAM practitioner because they often feel more listened to and respected by these practitioners than by their medical doctors, in part because of the amount of time they are able to spend with them. Whereas a typical followup visit with a rheumatologist may last fifteen or twenty minutes, a visit with a CAM practitioner might last thirty to forty-five minutes—a service for which you likely pay out of your own pocket. As well, people living with chronic illness are often frustrated with the failure of conventional medicine to provide a cure for their disease or help them get relief from their symptoms, and they fear the possible side effects of conventional medications.

In a 1999 study that looked at CAM use by people with osteoarthritis, fibromyalgia (a generalized aching condition that doesn't damage joints), and RA, almost half of the study participants:

- 87 percent of the participants said they used CAM to gain control of pain
- 86 percent used CAM because they heard it would help their condition
- 72 percent used CAM because they believed it to be harmless
- chiropractic and herbal therapies were two of the three most popular choices[15]

An alarming finding of this study was that 72 percent believed CAM to be harmless, which couldn't be farther from the truth—especially for people with RA. Consider the following risks.

Chiropractic

Traditional chiropractic medicine primarily focuses on manipulation of the spine. Because RA involves joint inflammation, stiffness, or joint instability, such spinal manipulation can damage joints. Thus, if you have RA, have inflammation, pain, or stiffness in your joints, it is essential that you never allow a chiropractor, *or anyone else* for that matter, to "adjust" your spine or other joints.

However, many chiropractors offer other types of treatment therapies besides spinal manipulation (such as ultrasound, electrical stimulation, vitamin and herbal therapies), but before visiting one, talk to your rheumatologist or GP. If you decide to try chiropractic treatment, make sure the practitioner holds a current license to practice all of the services they recommend during your visit.

Herbal Remedies and Supplements

The use of herbal remedies and supplements has skyrocketed. Many people believe that such remedies can prevent illness or disease, feel they are safer than conventional medications, or resort to them because they have difficulty getting in to see a doctor or are not comfortable with doctors.

While the public thinks herbal remedies and supplements are entirely safe, many have known toxicities, and in excessive dosages, can have significant side effects. So if you do choose to take herbal medicines, it is important for your safety to share this information with your rheumatologist and GP. Most will be happy to share with you their knowledge about herbal remedies and RA, and tell you about any scientific evidence proving or disproving their effectiveness. They also may be able to advise you about any known (and possibly dangerous) interactions with NSAIDs or disease management medications (DMMs) you are taking.

Approaching this topic with your doctors can be difficult, of course, because historically, western medical professionals have not taken herbal medicine seriously. You may fear they would look down on you for even considering this option. However, the opposite is more likely the case. Your doctor is bound to respect you for having open, honest communication with them and seeking their input on such an important decision.

If you are considering pregnancy, are pregnant, or are breast-feeding, use of herbal remedies is *not recommended*. Because herbal remedies are not regulated, there is simply no way of being assured that products are contaminate-free or correctly identified on the label. Some herbal products are known to cause spontaneous abortions. Older folks need to be careful too. As we age, our bodies have a decreased capacity to process the active ingredients in herbal remedies, and as a result, have a greater chance of experiencing side effects.

Below is an overview of the herbal remedies and supplements best known by the public, and often tried by people with RA. For in-depth information, refer to *The Arthritis Foundation's Guide to Alternative Therapies*. However, keep in mind that it is not specifically geared toward people with RA. You will need to read the text carefully to pull out the information that pertains to your disease.

BROMELAIN

An enzyme found in pineapple that is reported to help fight inflammation. No controlled studies have proven its effectiveness in RA.

CMO (*cetyl myristoleate*)

Sold as a supplement, CMO is one of a number of "natural" remedies reported to cure a number of types of arthritis: Ankylosing spondilitis, lupus, fibromyalgia, osteoarthritis, and RA, among others. No scientific evidence exists to support the claim (except for one study done in mice). It is *not recommended* for use in RA.

DEVIL'S CLAW (*harpagophytum procumbens*)

A plant from Africa used to treat inflammation and pain. It has not been scientifically proven effective in RA.

ECHINACEA (*echinacea purpurea*)

Primarily grown in the states of Washington and Oregon, Echinacea comes from a wildflower and is one of the biggest selling herbal remedies today. It is commonly used to "boost" the immune system to fight off colds or infection. Because the immune system in people with RA is already overactive, *echinacea is not recommended for use.*

FISH OIL (OMEGA-3 FATTY ACIDS)

See the section earlier in this chapter on Omega-3 fatty acids. These can be beneficial for people with RA.

FOLIC ACID

Methotrexate use reduces folate levels in the body. Studies show that taking 1 mg of folic acid daily[16] or 5 or 27.5 mg of folinic acid (Leucovorin®) weekly, ten hours following the methotrexate,[17] decreases side effects caused by the medication. Rheumatologists usually recommend trying folic acid first because it is sold over the counter and is considerably less expensive than the folinic acid, which must be prescribed.

GAMMA LINOLENIC ACID (GLA) (E.G., EVENING PRIMROSE OIL, BORAGE OIL)

There is strong scientific evidence showing that this omega-6 fatty acid has a positive effect against RA inflammation. However, talk to your rheumatologist before starting GLA supplements, as they do interact with RA medications such as NSAIDs.

GLUCOSAMINE

Touted as an "arthritis cure" several years ago, this supplement is used to treat the pain and stiffness caused by osteoarthritis—not RA. Unless or until several studies of glucosamine in large numbers of people with RA are reported, you are perhaps better off spending your health care dollars on therapies proven effective.

SELENIUM *(hypericum perforatum)*

Using this mineral, along with fish oil supplements, may help ease joint swelling and morning stiffness in RA. However, you only need a very small amount of selenium; excess dosages can be toxic, so check with your rheumatologist and GP before using.

ST. JOHN'S WORT *(hypricum perforatum)*

Although effective to treat the symptoms of depression, this herbal extract interacts with a number of drugs to decrease their effectiveness or increase their side effects. For instance, it makes cyclosporine less effective. It interacts with blood thinners, birth control pills, breathing medicines and other drugs to treat depression.

STINGING NETTLE (*urtica lioica*)

Reported to help fight inflammation and pain, but at present, no scientific studies have proven its effectiveness in RA.

THUNDER GOD VINE (*tripterygium wilfordii*)

The root of this Chinese herb has shown promise in uncontrolled studies as a disease management therapy for RA. Unlike other herbal and supplemental remedies, this one appears to have an effect on the disease itself, and not just the symptoms. Randomized, controlled studies in larger numbers of people with RA are needed to determine its place amongst traditional disease modifying medications. This herbal medicine has significant side effects, including the ability to reduce the blood counts and reduced fertility.

Following is a list of important things to remember or act on when using or considering CAM therapies:

> **Tell your physician that you are using or thinking about using CAM.** Most physicians today realize that CAM is here to stay and will not try to talk you out of using CAM therapies, unless they are likely to cause harm. Informing your rheumatologist and GP will help you to avoid dangerous interactions with medications, toxicities, or immune system boosting effects.
>
> **To date, there are no known "natural cures" for arthritis or RA.** Remember, "arthritis" is a word that represents over one hundred different diseases, most of which are vastly different from one another. A remedy that claims to treat all of them is highly unlikely to be a reliable one.
>
> **"Natural" doesn't always mean "safe."** Because the herbal remedy and supplement market is unregulated, products in these categories have not been tested for safety and effectiveness. Read the package carefully to determine the strength and purity of the active ingredient; these can vary greatly from manufacturer to manufacturer. Ask your rheumatologist and GP if they know of any reputable brands of the herbal remedy or supplement you are thinking about trying.
>
> **Research the pros and cons of CAM.**
> - When you research on the web or read written information about a given therapy, be careful to discern unbiased, valid information from product promotion. Sometimes the two look remarkably similar.
> - Search web-based medical databases (like Embase) for research studies on specific therapies you are considering; ask your local librarian for help.

- Call nonprofit organizations like The Arthritis Foundation (United States and Australia), The Arthritis Society (Canada), the Arthritis Foundation of New Zealand (Inc.), and Arthritis Care (United Kingdom) for information on CAM used for RA.
- Check with federal and local health regulatory agencies on licensing and regulation of CAM practitioners.

Ask these questions when evaluating information about CAM.

- what scientific evidence is there to support the therapy's methods, principles and effectiveness? Be sure to distinguish anecdotal evidence (such as personal testimonials) from controlled research studies. The latter deliver statistically valid results on which you can rely, whereas the former can be very misleading (there could, for example, be ten people who had adverse reactions for every one of the people who provided a glowing testimonial).
- does the therapy show effectiveness in treating RA in particular?
- What underlying theories, principles, or beliefs guide the therapy's understanding of health and illness. Do they mesh with your own?
- What kinds of procedures and techniques are you most likely to encounter?
- Does the therapy's approach exclude other forms of medicine?
- Are there any side effects with this type of therapy? How do they compare with conventional treatment?

Keep taking your DMM therapy when using CAM. Reports about herbal remedies or supplements being effective RA treatments pertain to helping with symptoms, *not controlling the underlying disease process.* Even if you have mild-to-moderate RA, DMM therapy is the only proven way to control the disease and delay or prevent joint damage and disability.

Try one CAM approach at a time. If you do decide to try CAM, start with only one therapy or remedy at a time (with your rheumatologist's and GP's knowledge) in combination with your DMM. Otherwise, you will not know which of the therapies is responsible for any changes, good or bad, in your symptoms.

Stop seeing any practitioner who:

- claims to offer a cure for RA or be able to perform a miracle
- doesn't give you enough information or show you published research into the risks or benefits of using the therapy they recommend
- looks down on you (or other practitioners) for using other health practices
- requires frequent, expensive visits

- insists that you use the practitioner's own (costly) products
- continues recommending the same therapy even after no significant change in your symptoms after three to six months
- makes you feel coerced (forced) into a treatment or therapy
- crosses your physical or emotional boundaries in a way that makes you feel uncomfortable[18]

Of course, these principles hold true for conventional medicine practitioners, health professionals and practitioners of complementary and alternative medicine alike.

Don't surrender to pressure. Friends, family, and store clerks are well intentioned when encouraging the use of CAM. However, most know little, if anything, about RA. You and your rheumatologist are the experts on your disease, and only you know how best to treat it. The correctness of your choices isn't up for debate with anyone who may be pressuring you; an effective response can be to politely thank them for their well-meaning advice, and let them know that you have a carefully thought-out treatment plan with an expert health-care team advising you every step of the way.

Chapter 7

THE MIND-BODY CONNECTION

"The real voyage of discovery consists
not in seeking new landscapes but in having new eyes."

—*Marcel Proust*

Browsing over the shelves of almost any bookstore, one discovers the myriad ways in which our attitudes, emotions, and thoughts are believed to influence our physical well-being. Popular writers such as Louise Hay, Bill Moyers, Bernie Seigal, Andrew Weil, and Deepak Chopra have taken mind-body ideas once considered fringe in the western hemisphere and brought them into our society's mainstream.

While some mind-body ideas are still considered far-fetched in western medical circles, others carry the stamp of approval that comes with rigorous scientific study. In fact, several fields of scientific research devote themselves solely to studying the relationship between the mind and the rest of the body. These include health psychology, biological psychiatry, and psychoneuroimmunology. A large amount of evidence indeed exists to support the notion that our mental states have a real effect on our physical well being.

By taking full advantage of the connection between mind and body, people with RA can directly influence their experience of the disease. For example, certain attitudes and personality attributes have been shown to be linked to decreased pain, less disability, and better overall health. And practice of mind-body techniques (such as yoga or guided imagery) is well documented to stimulate relaxation, which in turn is proven to aid sleep, decrease pain, and provide other health-related benefits.

Maximizing your mind-body connection is a vital aspect of your PLAN TO WIN. Unlike some aspects of living with the illness that are outside of your control, your feelings, beliefs, and attitudes are a unique and powerful area where *only you* have control.

In this chapter, we'll share examples of how other people with RA are coping well (and less well) with the mental and emotional aspects of living with chronic illness—and improving (or possibly worsening) their symptoms as a result. We'll explain the stages of grief, turmoil, and acceptance that many people experience when the disease strikes; then provide information about practices that use the mind to positively influence health.

MEDICINE AND THE MIND-BODY CONNECTION

The tides of medical opinion have swayed back and forth for decades over whether the mind does in fact influence health. Traditionally, western medical schools have operated on a biomedical foundation (meaning biology and medicine form the primary knowledge base), rather than taking into any serious account psychological and social factors.

Although researchers of mind-body therapies have not completely convinced the medical establishment of the effectiveness of these approaches, that is beginning to change—with new university-affiliated research centers devoted to this purpose and a new receptiveness on the part of medical doctors and scientists to take this research seriously.

Regardless, the majority of today's physicians and rheumatologists still think of mind-body practices as "alternative" medicine. Unfortunately, this label has the effect of invalidating mind-body practices and limiting the scope of their impact.[1]

We prefer to think of mind-body work not as an alternative to, but as an integral part of your PLAN TO WIN. Compelling research exists to show that mind-body approaches can assist with pain control, immune functioning, sleep, control of depression and anxiety, and can even indirectly influence the severity of your RA.

WHAT DOES THE RESEARCH SHOW?

Three types of research converge to lend credence to the idea that the way we think affects us physically: physiological research (which looks at biological and biochemical connections between the brain and the body); clinical studies (these test the effectiveness of mind-body practices on health outcomes); and epidemiological research (which looks for relationships between psychological influences and health outcomes in the general population).[2]

One field of investigation that may be of particular interest to people with RA is psychoneuroimmunology (PNI), which studies interactions among behavior, the nervous system, and the immune system. The roots of PNI sprouted in 1975, when researchers discovered that rats could be taught to modify their own immune functioning. The rats received flavored water containing a drug that suppressed their immunity. As expected, the animals developed an aversion to the flavor of the water. What was *unexpected* was that their immune functioning was also lower when they were exposed to the flavored water *without* the immunosuppressant drug in it. The rats' bodies expected the water to lower their immune system—and that expectation altered their immune functioning. Psychological forces *alone* were shown to suppress the animals' immune reactions.[3]

Since then, studies have repeatedly shown powerful links between what happens inside a human's mind and what happens in their body. For example:

- Women with advanced breast cancer who joined support groups in addition to using other medical interventions improved their quality of life *and* lived on average eighteen months longer than women who were not in support groups. This is longer than even cancer medications could have been expected to provide for the women at this advanced stage of cancer.[4]
- In the hours *before* patients received chemotherapy (a treatment which suppresses immune function and is often used for people with cancer), their immune functioning decreased. Here again, it was the psychological force of a learned association with a drug, rather than the drug itself, which had an impact.[5]
- People experiencing high levels of stress had fewer, and less effective, immune cells. For instance, students during the week of examinations; spouses of terminally ill partners, spouses caring for partners with dementia, and spouses going through marital problems or recovering from divorce.[6,7]
- Students who had more social contact and regularly practiced relaxation techniques had stronger immune functioning.[8]
- Individuals with higher levels of stress got more colds, respiratory infections, Esptein-Barr infections, and reactivation of the herpes virus.[9]

PERSONALITY AND HEALTH

Since the dawn of medicine, physicians have been noting relationships between psychological traits and health outcomes. This has been a mixed blessing. On the one hand, we have learned important information about personality traits that positively influence one's quality of life with chronic disease. On the other—and this is the rub—the information learned can be (and has been) used to blame people for having diseases in the first place; for instance, "It's because of your Type A personality that you have heart disease; it's because you're so stressed you got the flu; it's because you're so controlling you have XX." Clearly, this approach does not serve anyone; it is hard enough to live with a chronic illness without being told it is your own fault that you developed it, and that if you only had the right personality, attitudes, and beliefs, you could cure yourself.

But historically, this is what has happened to some people with RA, and you may even have been exposed to some of the folklore of that time. We offer a brief account of the historical information below, simply to help you arm yourself with knowledge in the event you are ever confronted with one of these outdated ideas during the course of your own journey with RA.

The Myth of the "Arthritic Personality"

Beginning in the 1920s and lasting until the 1970s, physicians attempted to define "the rheumatic personality," with the aim of being able to predict who might develop RA, and who was at high risk for development of more severe disease.[10]

During that period, rheumatoid arthritis was often described as a "classic psychosomatic disease," meaning the doctors considered the cause of the disease to be psychological, not physical. Physicians described people with RA as "full of passive-aggressive feelings, bitterness, self-pity and martyrdom; inhibited, masochistic, self-sacrificing, retiring and perfectionist;" and "more psychologically disturbed" than the general population. RA patients were said to have "unavailable emotions"; suffer from elevated hypochondriosis and hysteria, lack intelligence, have poor impulse control, poor ego strength, and a depressed mood not associated with physical pain. Females received a particular zing: they were viewed as suppressors of anger and sexuality.[11]

It is not surprising to find that the vast majority of these studies were methodologically flawed—for example, they failed to use control groups, and when control groups were used, conflicting results were found. There is, in fact, *no* evidence that rheumatic disease is more prevalent among the psychiatric population than among general population; indeed, there is a confirmed lower prevalence of RA in people with schizophrenia than in the general population.[12]

A more recent (1980s) study published in the *New England Journal of Medicine* found no link between personality traits and development of arthritis. Thus, today's doctors and researchers are convinced the idea of an "arthritic personality" is completely unfounded. The notion has been abandoned because there's no evidence that a certain type of personality is in place before RA onset that would in any way contribute to development of the disease.[13,14]

If it's any consolation, people with RA were not unique targets of harmful opinion. It was believed that schizophrenia was caused by bad mothering, and so on.

ATTITUDES AND ATTRIBUTES THAT SUPPORT HEALTH

Historical blunders aside, there are sound reasons to pay attention to information gleaned from mind-body research in more recent times. Over the past twenty years, a picture has formed of the attitudes and attributes of people who are coping best with arthritis and with other chronic diseases.

Information about health is rarely black and white, of course. Everyone has heard about Aunt Tilda, who smoked a pack a day until she got run over by a milk truck at the age of ninety-six. So, even if you embrace each of the helpful attributes described in this chapter, your RA may still be intractable. And should you have no desire to even read any further, let alone take this information seriously, your RA may improve or resolve itself completely (this can happen in about 10 percent of cases, in the early stages). And, of course, medical, social and environmental factors also play a critical role.

> **Mind-Body Ways to Support Optimal Health**
>
> - Control Pain
> - Pursue Emotional Wellness
> - Have a Positive Attitude
> - Ground Yourself in Reality
> - Experience Meaning in Life
> - Cope Actively
> - Maintain a Sense of Control
> - Believe in Yourself!

While it is possible to control aspects of one's thoughts, attitudes, and behavior, it's also important not to take on excessive psychological responsibility for your illness. It can lead to self-blame and self-criticism which surely will make you feel worse.[15]

With all of the warnings behind us, the following information is offered to show you the path taken by others in similar situations, where support and relief have been found. It all comes down to eight main factors: controlling pain; creating your own emotional wellness; maintaining a positive/optimistic attitude; staying grounded in reality; finding meaning in life and in having RA; coping actively rather than passively; maintaining a sense of control; and believing in yourself.

Controlling Pain

For most people with RA, pain is their number one disease-related challenge. In Chapter 2, we explained that RA pain is caused by inflammation or damage to joint tissues. Reversing inflammation and controlling tissue damage through medication, joint protection, and exercise is, therefore, essential to reducing pain. But unfortunately, even the most advanced medication therapy, combined with world-class physical therapy, devotion to exercise, and a strict diet, rarely succeeds in totally eliminating RA pain.

Pain is a complex issue that scientists are only just beginning to understand, and no two people experience it in exactly the same way. It is sometimes defined in strict physiological terms as an "an unpleasant sensory and

**Mind-Body Ways
to Support Optimal Health**

- **Control Pain**

- Pursue Emotional Wellness
- Have a Positive Attitude
- Ground Yourself in Reality
- Experience Meaning in Life
- Cope Actively
- Maintain a Sense of Control
- Believe in Yourself!

emotional experience arising from actual or potential tissue damage." This definition is lacking, though, because people with similar levels of tissue damage can have widely divergent experiences of pain. Pain can exist even where there is *no* tissue—for example, phantom limb pain (in which a person whose arm or leg has been amputated experiences painful sensations where their limb once was). By contrast, it's possible for someone to feel no pain at all when they've suffered significant physical trauma and are in shock (a soldier in battle is a good example).[16]

Although research has not established a relationship between pain and the course a person's RA will take over time, pain is a reliable predictor of the amount of medication you'll use; your own and your practitioners' assessments of your general health; your level of disability; and your future pain. Pain is also related to increased mental and emotional suffering. It can lead to feelings of pessimism, lessen one's ability to cope, and lead to a poor perception of one's own ability to function and manage symptoms.[17]

Clearly, it's essential to gain the upper hand on pain. Medication therapy provided by a rheumatologist or skilled doctor will go a long way. Physical therapy and joint protection also will help immensely. Therapeutic exercise and healthy living will do its fair share, and much of the remainder is up to your mind.

For example, we know beyond any doubt that stress, tension, and lack of sleep can make pain worse—all factors that are, to some degree, within an individual's mental control. The key is to use mental resources to break this cycle of pain. Practices that use the mind to influence the body (such as yoga, meditation, breathing, and emotional expressiveness) have been shown to bring stress levels down, loosen tension in the muscles, and lead to more restful sleep. Other approaches described later in this chapter (such as active coping and cognitive behavioral therapy) are also helpful in breaking the pain cycle.

Arthritis health professionals often recommend that people with RA use a scale from 1 to 10 to measure their pain before and after they begin a new practice or make changes in their daily life. By tracking changes in this way, you'll be able to clearly see what improves your pain, and what doesn't.

Several self-help books are available to assist with the mental aspects of pain control, including *The Relaxation Response* by Dr. Herbert Benson; *Pain: Learn to Live Without It*, by David Cory; and *The Arthritis Helpbook*, by Kate Lorig and James Fries.

Pursue Emotional Wellness

Emotional wellness has been shown to be one of the most important mental influences on health. Research shows that understanding your own feelings, accepting and expressing them (whether positive or negative), and doing work to release pent-up feelings such as anger, fear, self-blame, and the like, can go a long way toward enabling you to live a more pain-free, fulfilling life with RA.

In this section, we cover research and share helpful tips related to:

> **Mind-Body Ways to Support Optimal Health**
>
> • Control Pain
>
> • **Pursue Emotional Wellness**
>
> • Have a Positive Attitude
> • Ground Yourself in Reality
> • Experience Meaning in Life
> • Cope Actively
> • Maintain a Sense of Control
> • Believe in Yourself!

- emotional reactions to onset of RA
- emotional states such as depression, anxiety, and anger
- healthful expression of emotions

EMOTIONAL REACTIONS TO ONSET OF RA

Coming to grips with a chronic disease is, in real ways, like adjusting to the death of a loved one. You, too, may have suffered important losses. You might feel like you have lost your freedom from pain and disability, your financial security, or your feeling of control over your life. It could feel as though you lost your independence, your self-esteem, your happiness, your hope ... the list could no doubt be lengthened by every reader of this book.

Like the passing of someone you care about, adjusting to RA presents an enormous emotional challenge. Losing one's ability to do certain things is extremely difficult to accept. If that weren't enough all on its own, disability is often compounded by problems with work, family, money, and simply accomplishing the things we need to in a day. Add chronic pain and unpredictable flareups, and it's obvious why people with RA often feel a loss of control and a sense of powerlessness.

Losing some of your independence—or feeling as though you have—can be devastating. So can living with uncertainty: How bad will this disease get? How can I possibly handle this on my own? How will I find my way around the unfamiliar medical system? Will I lose my job? Will my child get RA? Will my joints become deformed? Does RA mean I am going to die earlier?

These intense feelings of loss, powerlessness, and uncertainty are not unique to people with RA—they are experienced by people with a wide range of chronic illnesses. Like mourning for a loved one, it's natural (and helpful) to react to chronic illness by moving through a range of feelings similar to what a person experiences when they lose a loved one, including shock, fear, anger, despair, and eventually acceptance—sometimes in this order, oftentimes not.

The explanation below is typically used to help people understand the grieving process. We offer it here as broad guidance for understanding your emotional reactions to having RA. The stages suggest a sequence of reactions but, in reality, people mourn in a variety of ways. Feelings such as anger may appear to be resolved, only to surface again at a later time. Or you might go through the stages in a different order.

Shock and disbelief

When your doctor or rheumatologist explained your diagnosis, you might have felt numb or empty, or perhaps you felt nothing at all. Maybe you experienced a sense of denial: "There must be some mistake"; "I knew I didn't trust this doctor"; or something similar. These feelings of shock and disbelief typically last from several days to several weeks, although it's not uncommon to be struck with disbelief for moments or during certain periods of one's life even years later.

Searching, anxiety, and fear

Blaming and anger are common during this stage, as you search for cause and meaning in the fact that you now have RA. The feelings can be directed outwardly in the form of blame, "If only my spouse hadn't lost his job and brought so much stress on me," or inwardly as guilt, "Why is God punishing me?"

Anxiety and fear can lead to crying, insomnia, difficulty concentrating, racing heart, diarrhea, vomiting, sweating, startling easily, and changes in appetite. This stage often lasts from the second week to the fourth or fifth month after loss. Some people use this stage to their advantage, channeling their energy toward gathering all the information they can get about RA. If you can do so, all the better. Understanding arthritis will take you a long way toward achieving your optimal health.

Disorganization, despair, and depression

These feelings frequently follow the full realization of one's diagnosis. It's hard to accomplish normal activities during this time—for emotional reasons, in addition to the painful challenges posed by your RA. You might feel as though you are simply "going through the motions" of life. You could be overwhelmed by sadness or a sense of futility. You might withdraw from friends and loved ones, feel restless, or be preoccupied with the disease. Marital problems are also common during this stressful time. If that's you, we encourage you and your life partner to read Chapter 7.

People who are depressed typically experience symptoms such as insomnia (trouble getting to sleep, waking up in the middle of the night or early morning, and not being able to get back to sleep), changes in eating patterns, lack of enjoyment of anything, suicidal feelings, and feelings of hopelessness. If you are experiencing these symptoms, please talk to your doctor or rheumatologist as soon as possible. We also recommend that you read the "Depression" and "Anxiety" sections below.

Reorganization

Eventually, preoccupation with the disease passes, and life regains fuller meaning. You are able to interact once again with others, and to plan for the future. You might still be overwhelmed by sadness from time to time, but it goes away. The RA diagnosis has been integrated into your life, but is no longer the emotional center of your life.[18]

EMOTIONAL STATES: DEPRESSION AND ANXIETY

Emotional states such as depression, anxiety, and anger are understandable and common reactions to living with a chronic disease. However, remaining stuck in such emotional states over long periods can negatively affect your overall wellness, including having a detrimental effect on your RA.

You might feel trapped when you learn about the detrimental effects these emotional states can have on your body, and potentially fall into blaming yourself: for instance, "I'm making myself sicker by being so depressed about being sick!" However, as we've said before, such blaming is only destructive—and anyone who tries it on you should be told so (see the section on emotional expression).

The information presented here is based on the following well-documented fact: people with RA typically experience psychological distress. We present it because of another well-documented fact: the way you manage that stress can affect your level of pain, disability and further distress. The more information at your fingertips, the more power you have to improve your quality of life—both now and in the future.

Depression

People who are depressed typically feel hopeless, have less energy, suffer from low self esteem, have difficulty concentrating or making decisions, experience changes in their patterns of eating and sleeping, lose or gain weight, and sometimes cry more easily or have suicidal thoughts.

Depression can occur in reaction to loss (such as the losses posed by RA) or some other external event; it also can occur in the absence of an external trigger. Some medications used in the treatment of RA (such as prednisone and, more rarely, some NSAIDs) can also produce depression as a side effect.[19]

Studies estimate that up to 50 percent of people with RA are depressed,[20] and about 17 percent have major depressive disorder. This level is higher than that seen in the general population, but similar to the level of depression found among people living with other chronic medical conditions.[21,22,23,24]

Estimates of the level of depression among people with RA are sometimes falsely inflated because depression questionnaires contain items assessing symptoms such as fatigue and sleep disturbance, which are direct manifestations of RA, and not necessarily indicative of depression.[25] Although the level of depression in people with RA is higher than the general population, it's worthwhile noting the majority of people with RA are *not* depressed.

A link does not appear to exist between the severity of RA or RA-related pain and whether an individual becomes depressed. However, other factors are clearly associated with development of depression in people with RA, such as lack of social support, high amounts of daily stress, insufficient money, lack of confidence in one's ability to cope, loss of independence, and how long one has had RA (a longer time living with the disease predicts higher likelihood of depression).

Depression can lead you to hold a poorer view of your own health and your physical abilities,[26] which can, unfortunately, become a self-fulfilling prophecy (in studies, a poor view of one's own health and abilities has, in fact, been linked to poorer health outcomes).

Often, people who are depressed either don't want to be around others or simply can't bring themselves to get out of bed or leave their residence, leading to social isolation and often to loss of employment and financial difficulties as well. One four-year study of people with RA found that depressed individuals spent 5.8 more days in bed per month than did their nondepressed counterparts.

Once depressed, people have a tendency to perceive their own health and physical abilities in an even more negative light than is actually the case.[27]

Anxiety

Anxiety is characterized by persistent worry, restlessness, easy fatigue, changes in sleep patterns, muscle tension, irritability, and difficulty concentrating. Few studies distinguish anxiety from depression. Those that do have found elevated levels of anxiety in people with RA—In one well-controlled study, people with RA were found to be four times more likely to be anxious than control subjects.[28,29,30] Again, many characteristics of anxiety are also symptoms of RA, so this number may be inflated. Because of these overlapping symptoms, anxiety can be difficult to detect in people with RA. And, of course, effectively treating the RA and reducing its symptoms can lead to improvements in anxiety.

Treatment for depression and anxiety

The good news is that depression and anxiety can in many cases be prevented. By learning all that you can about the disease (and having your loved ones learn as much as they can), you can gain a sense of control and support, and ward off feelings of hopelessness. Early, aggressive medical treatment leading to control of the disease means you'll experience less pain, fatigue, and disability—which, in turn, will make you less likely to have reason to become depressed in the first place.

Clinical depression, whether or not it is associated with chronic illness, is highly treatable. Studies show that for people with RA, antidepressants reduce pain independently of improving mood.[31] The mechanism for this is not precisely known, but it is presumed that antidepressants cause positive changes in sleep patterns, relaxation of tense muscles, or possibly an analgesic effect explained by an underlying common neurochemical pathway.[32,33] What's more, most people report improved functional ability with antidepressants.[34] No serious interaction problems are known to exist between antidepressants and medications typically used to treat RA.[35] For people with anxiety, pharmacological treatments known as anxiolytics are available. A nonaddictive one is Buspirone.

Untreated, depression can result in:

- an increase in your pain and other symptoms of RA
- a decrease in the amount of your self-care
- a decrease in your motivation to adhere to your treatment plan
- a direct negative impact on the RA itself[36]
- decreased immune functioning due to manifestations of depression such as changes in diet, sleep, and activity[37]
- greater physical symptoms such as fatigue, pain, and sleep disturbances—which may lead doctors to change the medical treatment and increase medication to levels greater than actually required to treat the disease[38]

Studies show that physicians fail to recognize depression in their non-hospitalized patients at least 50 percent of the time (either because depressive symptoms overlap with symptoms of RA, or due to a lack of physician knowledge or assessment skills).[39] If you think you are depressed, but your general practitioner or rheumatologist has not diagnosed you as such, be proactive. Tell your physician you think you may be depressed and would benefit from antidepressant medication; or see another qualified professional.

Try not to accept depression, anxiety, or anger as a chronic (ongoing) way of feeling—learn as much as you can about why you are feeling this way, and obtain professional support and help from family and friends to bring about change in this area of your life. The positive effects on your disease will be well worth the effort you invest.

EMOTIONAL EXPRESSIVENESS

How many times were you told as a child that if you don't have anything nice to say, you shouldn't say anything at all? Apparently, well-intended advice such as this did many of us more harm than good. Expressing our feelings, both positive and negative, has proven healthful effects.

Consider this:

- One study asked women who were about to have biopsies for potential breast cancer to complete a questionnaire about emotional expressiveness. Women whose biopsies later turned out to be malignant (meaning cancerous) were significantly more likely to have indicated on the questionnaire that they rarely expressed anger.[40]

- In an investigation of people with RA, one group was assigned to write about neutral topics; the other group wrote about the most stressful event of their lives. Participants were examined prior to the writing, two weeks later, two months later, and four months later. RA patients who wrote about their most stressful experiences showed a significant improvement in overall disease activity that was still evident four months after the writing exercise.[41]

- In another study, subjects with RA who accepted the emotional significance of their illness had better health outcomes over three years than those who denied its significance.[42]

- A recent study of people with RA who underwent an intervention that induced an hour of mirthful laughter in them showed a direct, immediate, positive response in their immune systems, compared to people in a control group who did not laugh for the hour.[43]

- In chronic pain research, certain ways of handling anger have been associated with greater pain. The research suggests that people who suppress anger or express it through hostility are more prevalent among chronic pain populations.[44]

- In cardiovascular research, high levels of hostility have been linked to increased coronary disease and mortality. For example, in a study which included a twenty-five-year follow-up, 14 percent of doctors and 20 percent of lawyers at age twenty-five with high hostility scores were dead by age fifty; whereas only 2 percent of doctors and 4 percent of lawyers with low hostility scores were dead by that age.[45]

- In one study of people with RA, those who had high levels of hostility had poorer health outcomes three years later than those who had low levels of hostility.[46]

Do you find that you let out your feelings at times when you really don't want to? What about expressing your emotions, then later regretting that you did? This kind of "emotional ambivalence" is linked with lower psychological well-being in the general public and in people with RA.[47]

For help learning to recognize and express your feelings, consider reading *Opening Up: The Healing Power of Confiding in Others* by James Pennebaker (1990) or *The Dance of Anger: A Woman's Guide to Changing the Patterns of Intimate Relationships* by Harriet Lerner (1997). You also might consider establishing a relationship with a psychologist or other qualified therapist with whom you can safely let out your feelings. (See Chapter 3 for help finding your personal best fit with a therapist.) Or, if group work and social interaction appeals to you, you might wish to try attending a support group or the Arthritis Self Management Program (North America) or Challenging Arthritis (United Kingdom). Another option is to make a concerted effort to share all of your feelings with just one person to start with—say, your spouse or a good friend. (It's a good idea to tell them ahead of time that you're planning this new approach, and to ask for their support and involvement. For other communication-related tips, see Chapter 8.)

Maintaining A Positive Attitude

Can a positive attitude truly affect your health? Yes—in several concrete ways, actually. A positive attitude:

- acts directly on your immune system, hormonal system, and cardiovascular system—For example, the neurotransmitters released when we're happy have been shown to affect our immune systems in a positive way
- increases the likelihood that you'll engage in health-promoting behaviors like exercising, eating well, and following your health providers' advice
- increases the likelihood that you'll get support from friends, loved ones, and the community at large.[48]

> **Mind-Body Ways to Support Optimal Health**
>
> - Control Pain
> - Pursue Emotional Wellness
> - **Have a Positive Attitude**
> - Ground Yourself in Reality
> - Experience Meaning in Life
> - Cope Actively
> - Maintain a Sense of Control
> - Believe in Yourself!

Optimism can be thought of as the degree to which you expect your future to be positive versus negative, or as a style of explaining to yourself the events that happen in your life. For instance, do you blame yourself for negative events ("I'm a bad person, which is why I didn't get the promotion"), or see the cause of such an event as something more neutral ("It just wasn't

the right time for me to get the promotion")? Or do you turn it into a positive ("I'm glad I didn't get it, because it means something better must be
out there waiting for me")? Do you see the meaning of negative events in
terms of "forever," or in terms of "right now" ("I'm going to be disabled for
the rest of my life" versus "The RA symptoms might improve a lot if I set
goals and stick with my treatment program")?

Whether an individual is optimistic or pessimistic appears to have a
strong influence upon their health outcomes. In a study that followed men
for thirty-five years, those with an optimistic personality style when first
tested were healthier *thirty-five years later* than those with a pessimistic
style,[49] and those with cardiac diseases had longer survival times than their
less optimistic counterparts.[50] In another study, women with breast cancer
who were determined to have a "fighting spirit" versus those who felt hopeless about their disease were more likely to outlive their counterparts at five,
ten, and fifteen year follow-ups.[51] Other studies show people who are optimistic have fewer days of illness and fewer physician visits, recover more
quickly and fully after surgery, and have stronger immune systems. People
who experienced surprise, joy, and interest experienced less pain and depression.[52] People who tended to be distrustful of others and the world were
shown to be at greater risk for morbidity (from all causes) and mortality.[53]

One of the few optimism studies conducted specifically with people who
have RA revealed similar findings: those who expressed negative or exag-
gerated interpretations of their illness were more depressed and disabled
than those whose beliefs were more positive.[54]

If you find that you have a tendency to be more negative than optimistic,
take heart: Optimism is something you can actually *learn* if you wish to,
through cognitive behavioral therapy (consult a registered psychologist for
information).

Staying Grounded in Reality

Research shows that people with RA who
use distortions in the way they think (*cognitive distortions*, as psychologists call
them) tend to be more depressed and experience more pain and physical distress.
Everyone uses cognitive distortions from
time to time, but when they become a consistent way of thinking, such distortions
can become quite destructive.

Examples of cognitive distortions best
avoided are:

- *personalization*: feeling that you are
  responsible for negative occurrences

> **Mind-Body Ways
> to Support Optimal Health**
>
> - Control Pain
> - Pursue Emotional Wellness
> - Have a Positive Attitude
>
> - **Ground Yourself in Reality**
>
> - Experience Meaning in Life
> - Cope Actively
> - Maintain a Sense of Control
> - Believe in Yourself!

- *overgeneralization*: thinking that one negative outcome predicts other negative outcomes
- *selective abstraction*: focusing on negative aspects of situations to the exclusion of positive aspects
- *catastrophizing*: expecting the outcome of an event to be a catastrophe

People with RA who are more reality-oriented, believe in themselves, and are involved in proactively managing their disease have less psychological and physical distress as a result of their disease.[55]

If you recognize cognitive distortions as something you do a lot of, you might consider seeing a psychologist for cognitive therapy, which focuses on helping people change their thinking styles.

Experiencing Meaning in Life

An analysis of over eight hundred people with RA found those who had a strong "sense of coherence" (meaning they believed that the circumstances in their life made sense, that life itself made sense; and that there was enough meaning in life to justify the effort and energy required to face life's challenges) were in better overall health, had less difficulty with day-to-day activities, less pain, and less feelings of helplessness, regardless of the severity of their disease.[56]

Another recent study found that people with a strong sense of coherence were less depressed and anxious, reported higher levels of well-being, and experienced less functional disability.[57]

> **Mind-Body Ways to Support Optimal Health**
>
> - Control Pain
> - Pursue Emotional Wellness
> - Have a Positive Attitude
> - Ground Yourself in Reality
>
> - **Experience Meaning in Life**
>
> - Cope Actively
> - Maintain a Sense of Control
> - Believe in Yourself!

Similarly, a 1998 study found that people with RA who had a low sense of coherence experienced more depression and pain.[58]

If you don't already experience meaning in your life, how does one find such meaning? Practicing religion or cultivating a spiritual attitude— whether formally through an organization or alone through reading, prayer, meditation, or the like—is the path taken by some. Faith and prayer have been shown to help people cope with chronic illness, and are associated with positive physical outcomes. Others work with a therapist or explore meaning through art or other forms of creative expression. Whatever practice works best for you is the perfect one—and all the better if you have support in doing so.

Coping Actively

Mind-Body Ways to Support Optimal Health
• Control Pain
• Pursue Emotional Wellness
• Have a Positive Attitude
• Ground Yourself in Reality
• Experience Meaning in Life
• **Cope Actively**
• Maintain a Sense of Control
• Believe in Yourself!

Most of us don't think much about *how* we cope with life's challenges ... we just cope.

Surprisingly, a substantial body of research has been dedicated to looking at the *ways* in which people cope. Researchers found that people who *actively* cope with life's demands fare better than those who cope *passively*. They function better psychologically and physically, and experience less depression.[59]

By "actively coping," they mean that a person focuses directly on their problem; actively seeks to solve or relieve it; and takes on personal responsibility for doing so. Ways that people cope actively with RA include:

- seeking information about the disease and its treatment
- diverting attention away from pain (through practices such as relaxation, guided imagery, changing thought processes; or activities such as reading, artwork, or socializing)
- alternating periods of rest with periods of activity
- adapting the physical environment at work and home
- taking steps to control pain (breaking the pain cycle; exercising; following the advice of rheumatologists and health practitioners)
- cognitive restructuring (reframing negative things into positive; "fixing" cognitive distortions; looking on the sunny side)

"Passive coping," by contrast, occurs when a person:

- does not seek a solution
- denies the problem
- gives up control to external forces
- withdraws; escapes into fantasy; distances from the situation
- blames others or oneself for the problem
- passively accepts a situation

This type of passive coping includes any way of reacting that avoids confronting one's problems squarely. For example, in passive coping, one might:

- avoid seeing the rheumatologist because of embarrassment or guilt about admitting missed doses of medications

- ignore feelings by focusing on something else—for example, rather than acknowledging feelings of anger toward a friend who pushed unsolicited advice about "curing" RA, one might focus on gossiping with them about an acquaintance
- avoid emotions (eating instead of feeling lonely; drinking instead of feeling anxious; choosing to feel numb in life instead of experiencing the range of emotions beneath the surface)[60]

According to research, this type of passive coping can be hazardous to your well-being. There's remarkable consensus that passive coping strategies are associated with poorer adjustment, lower self-esteem, and greater depression. This is true both in the general population and in people with RA.[61]

Some passive coping strategies not only don't help, but are associated with greater pain, greater functional disability and a lesser ability to cope with life. These include: catastrophizing (expecting the outcome of an event to be a catastrophe), wishful thinking, avoidance behaviors and fear-avoidance beliefs (reducing physical activity and exercise, withdrawing from social activities, stopping work, avoiding unpleasant obligations such as work, chores, relationships). These may be useful short-term strategies in a crisis—such as in the initial stages of diagnosis—but over the long term can result in the above negative outcomes, in addition to feelings of loss of control and pessimistic beliefs about your own capabilities.[62,63] With poor coping strategies, you may not be able to take good care of yourself and may generalize feelings of not being able to cope to other aspects of your life.

Switching from passive to active coping is definitely easier said than done. Most people spend a lifetime learning and perfecting ways of protecting themselves from painful feelings and difficult situations. People use passive coping strategies to great effect in avoiding strong and uncomfortable emotions. What most people don't realize is that these strategies don't work in the long run—because emotions have an uncanny way of resurfacing in different places and in different ways. An argument could even be made, based on the RA research, that they surface through increased pain and disability.

To switch into active coping, emotions must be felt, acknowledged, and worked through. Feelings can be expressed in any way that feels right for you: through writing, song, movement, artwork or verbal expression. Many people find the most powerful way of working through feelings is by having them "witnessed" by another person of their choosing—spouse, friend, therapist. Whichever outlet you choose, you'll be making a strong contribution to your optimal health.

Maintaining A Sense of Control

Mind-Body Ways to Support Optimal Health
• Control Pain
• Pursue Emotional Wellness
• Have a Positive Attitude
• Ground Yourself in Reality
• Experience Meaning in Life
• Cope Actively
• **Maintain a Sense of Control**
• Believe in Yourself!

Having a sense of control over one's life is important to pretty much anyone. Research shows that, in general, it's associated with higher quality of life and increased longevity (length of life).[64]

For people with RA, possessing a sense of control is linked with beneficial health effects[65] such as positive mood, better psychological functioning and adjustment,[66] and decreased disability and pain.[67] Conversely, experiencing hopelessness and lack of control is related to poor health prognoses in people diagnosed with various diseases.[68]

At the time of RA onset, it's common for people to feel like their control has gone out the window—especially in the very early stages. You may feel you've lost control over your daily life (as a result of unpredictable flares and symptoms); over the shape that your future will take; over your ability to do your job, among other losses. The more you learn about the disease and its management, though, the more obvious it will become to you that *your* choices and behaviors can greatly influence the impact of your disease—and the stronger your feelings of hope and control will become.

Learned helplessness is the opposite of having a sense of control. It's a feeling that one is without any control over the negative events happening to them—resulting in a sense of powerlessness and hopelessness. A scale called the "Arthritis Helplessness Index" showed that people with high degrees of this feeling experienced more psychological distress (such as depression and anxiety) and more physical disability (such as pain and greater day-to-day difficulties with the disease), and tended to use passive coping styles.[69]

Stress can also make you feel out of control—it feels as though life is somewhat unpredictable, overwhelming, and uncontrollable. Research shows that when a person feels they have some control over their stressors, the impact of that stress on their immune system is mediated.[70] Our conclusion: This is yet one more excellent reason to actively manage your stress levels. Be realistic about how much you can take on; practice saying no; care less about what other people think; and invite loved ones or a professional to support you in making changes in these areas. It also can be beneficial to join a mind-body awareness program, where you'll not only learn to recognize your body's signs of stress (such as changes in muscle tension, heart rate, breathing rate, sweating) but also learn how to regulate these responses.

If the above descriptions of stress, helplessness, and absence of control apply to you, it may be helpful to try to adopt the belief that you *can* influence your own health. Research has found that people with this "internal locus of control" have more positive psychological and physical functioning, and report less pain and depression, regardless of disease severity.[71] Of course, it's essential not to take this to the extreme of blaming yourself for the illness or the fact that it is not cured! And, if stress is a significant factor for you, give serious consideration to learning and practicing a relaxation technique (more on this later).[72]

Maintaining a sense of control is, of course, different (and much more positive for health) than wanting to control everything and believing one *can* control everything. This is part of what's been described as "Type A" behavior—exerting social control and dominance over others; it leads to greater risk for illness.[73]

What can you do to regain or maintain a healthy sense of control?

One of the best ways is to decide that you are going to create a health plan, which is what this book is all about: getting information and making informed choices, taking care of your body and spirit to the best of your ability, and getting help with all of it as need may dictate.

Another option is participating in a self-management course offered through your local arthritis organization. The Arthritis Self-Management Program (ASMP) is offered in thousands of North American communities through The Arthritis Foundation in the USA and The Arthritis Society in Canada. In the United Kingdom, the same program is offered under a different name: Challenging Arthritis.

Although the program is not aimed specifically toward the needs of people with RA, in general, ASMP participants benefit not only by increasing their knowledge, but by increasing their confidence in their ability to cope with their disease.[74] Participants also report decreased levels of pain and better psychosocial functioning.[75] If a group setting appeals to you, and no RA-specific group is available, you may wish to give ASMP a try.

Believing In Yourself

Another seemingly obvious but helpful attitude to adopt is *believing in yourself*. It has been shown in research that a person's "self-efficacy" (their beliefs about their own capabilities) affects whether they initiate and persist with behaviors that will help their condition (such as exercising, sticking with their medication therapy, keeping a health journal, etc.).

The "Arthritis Self-Efficacy Scale" measures an individual's belief in their ability to

Mind-Body Ways to Support Optimal Health
• Control Pain
• Pursue Emotional Wellness
• Have a Positive Attitude
• Ground Yourself in Reality
• Experience Meaning in Life
• Cope Actively
• Maintain a Sense of Control
• **Believe in Yourself!**

perform basic activities and manage pain. As might be expected, when tested on this scale, people who believed in their own abilities were found to have less depression, pain, and perceived disability—regardless of how active their disease was.

INTEGRATING HELPFUL ATTITUDES AND ATTRIBUTES INTO YOUR LIFE

As we've seen, people who work toward their own emotional wellness tend to have a much better experience of living with RA than those who don't.

Adopting these approaches can be hard work, however, since most of us have spent our lives developing extremely effective strategies and defenses for shutting down our feelings and avoiding challenging emotional territory. With dedication to this type of personal development, things like emotional expressiveness can, over time, become second-nature to us. Most people find the work pays off in many ways, in addition to improving symptoms of RA—such as in stronger relationships and greater fulfillment in life in general.

This chapter has merely scratched the surface of all the ways to use your mind's connection with your body to optimal advantage in managing your RA. We encourage you to read more on the subject, and also to explore mind-body practices that appeal to you.

PRACTICES THAT SUPPORT A MIND-BODY APPROACH TO HEALTH

It takes persistence, hard work, and the assistance of a knowledgeable group of people or practitioners to develop the personal attitudes and attributes shown to support optimal health. Practicing mind-body techniques can also be very helpful in this regard.

Relaxation

A large body of information exists to demonstrate the therapeutic effect of relaxation on health. For example:

- when a person relaxes, her heart and breathing rates slow down, and her blood pressure becomes lower
- relaxation helps people change their emotional reactions when dealing with unavoidable problems[76]
- regular states of relaxation make the body less susceptible to the effects of stress.[77] As we have seen, this is important for people with RA, since stress is known to add to tension, feelings of loss of control, and increased pain

- relaxation also has been shown to decrease pain and disability[78,79,80,81] and boost the immune system.[82,83] Relaxation via mindfulness training for people with chronic pain (not specifically RA) showed a 72 percent decrease in pain, and people reduced their pain overall by 33 percent; results still held at eighteen months follow-up

Practices found to elicit the relaxation response are meditation, yoga, biofeedback, progressive relaxation, guided imagery, and hypnosis.[84]

With such compelling evidence, we do encourage you to learn a relaxation technique that you enjoy, and get in the habit of practicing it twice a day if you can manage it (or more if you get addicted to the peaceful feeling!). If you find it hard to make the time or to keep practicing, join a group to support your practice or see a practitioner as often as your finances allow.

Cognitive Behavioral Therapy

This type of therapy, practiced by trained psychologists, is based on the idea that pain and symptoms are influenced by a person's cognition (thinking) and their behavioral response to their illness. As such, the goal with this therapy is to help individuals change their thoughts and actions in response to their disease symptoms.[85]

A large amount of research has been dedicated to exploring the effectiveness of cognitive behavioral therapy for people with RA:

- treatments that included relaxation, coping skills, and cognitive restructuring (reframing thoughts) demonstrated a significant positive impact in reducing pain, depression, and anxiety, and increasing use of adaptive coping strategies[86,87] in people with RA.[88,89,90]

- improved sleep, improved adherence to exercise programs, reduced functional impairment, and decreased joint involvement[91] also have been shown to be improved by cognitive behavioral therapy, but results are less consistent.[92]

Professionals who practice cognitive behavioral therapy use three main strategies to help people control pain and symptoms:

1. Concentrative attention: The individual focuses on one object or sensation to the exclusion of everything else.
2. Mindful awareness: The individual does not focus on any object or thought; instead, they remain open to each new thought or sensation as it arises.

3. Focus on sensations: The individual focuses on the sensations themselves, without interpretation or judgment (for example, whether something hurts or is uncomfortable).[93]

Clients usually learn one or a combination of these techniques: relaxation, biofeedback, active coping strategies (such as alternating periods of rest and activity), understanding common cognitive distortions (as described earlier in this chapter under "Staying Grounded in Reality"), and rational thought replacement (for instance, replacing "never" and "always" in thoughts with "sometimes" or "right now.")[94]

If cognitive behavioral therapy appeals to you, ask your rheumatologist or other people you trust for names of good local psychologists, or consult your telephone directory under "psychologists." Some therapists practice this type of work and others don't: call to ask before you set up an appointment.

Getting Support

Like eating well and exercising, support is essential to optimal health for all people—whether they have RA or not.

In research with healthy individuals and those with a range of acute and chronic illnesses, greater amounts of social support have been associated with lowered risk of morbidity and early death; improved immune, psychological, and social functioning; decreased depression[95] and enhanced recovery.[96] Conversely, lack of social support has been linked with impaired immune functioning[97] and depression.[98] The relationship between social isolation and early death is actually as strong statistically as the relationship between early death and smoking or high cholesterol.[99]

In people with RA, those receiving more social support experience higher self-esteem, greater ability to function independently, better psychological adjustment and life satisfaction, greater ability to meet life's demands, decreased negative affect after undesirable events,[100] and less depression.[101,102]

Clearly, getting support is a vital aspect of your PLAN TO WIN. There are many forms of support that can be valuable—some come from friends and loved ones, others are provided by health professionals or support groups.

With emotional support, one feels loved or cared for. Positive regard is another type of support: When someone holds you in high regard, it provides important acknowledgment that your beliefs and feelings are valid. Other types of support include provision of information about RA, physical assistance, financial support, and companionship. Even pets can provide helpful support—they've been shown to positively impact health.[103]

As described in Chapter 7, people with RA report feeling most supported when they are able to express feelings and concerns, when they receive hope and encouragement, and when they are given *asked-for* information and advice. They express most satisfaction when getting emotional support from a spouse or partner, and more tangible support—such as helpful medications and pain management tips—from health professionals.

People with RA describe unhelpful support as anything that minimizes the severity of their illness. In addition, forcing cheerfulness; avoiding the person with RA; avoiding discussion of the illness; and being overly solicitous or pitying also were found to be unhelpful. Lack of emotional support from a spouse, ineffective help from health professionals, and unwanted or unsolicited advice from friends are all cited as unhelpful.

Although formal groups exist to provide support to people with a range of special interests (for instance, women's groups, spiritual groups, men's groups, chronic pain groups, arthritis support groups), a "support group" also can consist of a network of friends and family you care about.

A few studies also have been published on the effectiveness of support groups for people with RA. These reported positive outcomes but were flawed by lack of control groups.[104] If joining a support group for people with arthritis appeals to you, contact your local office of The Arthritis Society or Arthritis Foundation—there's a good chance one exists in your community. If not, consider other types of support groups—your local health or recreation center may have information about what's available nearby.

Guided Imagery

Not much well-designed research exists to demonstrate the effectiveness of guided imagery on its own—it is often used in conjunction with relaxation, hypnosis, or in therapy. One study of people with RA that compared medical treatment alone, with a relaxation group, and with a hypnosis and imagery group found the hypnosis and imagery group to show the most improvements in symptoms and disease activity.[105] A few articles in scientific journals have described improvement in one person with RA after treatment with imagery.

A guided imagery session typically begins with a relaxation exercise or with induction of a hypnotic state ("hypnosis" is the induction of a particular state of mind, while "imagery" is an activity). The individual imagines seeing something in particular (although "seeing" can be substituted with or enhanced by a feeling, sound, or smell).

Visualization

In visualization, a person is either guided by a practitioner or learns to guide herself through relaxation and then a series of images to promote healing. For example, a person with cancer might visualize a discussion with the cancer cells to ascertain what practices would promote healing. Remarkable success has been reported with this technique in many otherwise untreatable conditions, although no specific research has been done on people with RA.

Medical Hypnosis

People can be taught self-hypnosis, which is a technique of concentration that enables the person to induce relaxation or control some of their body's functions. Although no research exists specifically on medical hypnosis in people with RA, it has been demonstrated to be successful in reducing pain and anxiety, and in increasing a sense of control in people with a range of health problems.[106]

Biofeedback

Biofeedback is a technique in which a person's body parameter (such as heart rate) is measured and amplified to provide information for them about their body's processes. The person observes patterns of rises and falls in the heart rate, and is taught techniques (such as breathing and visualization) that alter the rate. Great success has been made in teaching people to control otherwise unconscious body patterns through biofeedback techniques.

Psychotherapy

Based on compelling information about the usefulness of emotional expression in creating health, it seems like a natural extension to assume that psychotherapy (talking with a trained psychologist to explore thoughts and emotions) would be useful for people with RA, and this is likely the case. At this point, however, there have only been a few studies investigating the impact of individual therapy on people with RA. These studies did report positive health benefits, but were methodologically flawed, making it difficult to draw firm conclusions about the efficacy of this type of treatment for people with RA. However, it seems unlikely that it could cause harm, and at minimum it could help with the emotional challenges that can accompany the disease.

One excellent study of the effects of psychotherapy on women with metastatic breast cancer who were randomly assigned to supportive group psychotherapy did show a positive effect: The women lived an average of eighteen months longer than their matched controls who did not attend such a support group. Four years later, none of the women who had been in the control group (those who did not attend a support group) were alive, yet one-third of the women who had been in the support group were still alive.[107]

Choosing The Best Practice For You

With so many choices of mind-body practices, it can be hard to know where to begin. Our best advice is to choose a practice that appeals to you—

one that you can afford; that offers the amount of social interaction you prefer (from very little to quite a lot); and that is provided by a trained practitioner with whom you feel comfortable and whom you trust.

If it helps you to compare the effectiveness of some of these mind-body practices, three excellent studies done with people with RA demonstrated the following:

1. Biofeedback and relaxation were more effective in pain relief than no treatment.
2. Biofeedback, relaxation, and cognitive behavioral therapy were superior to social support groups and no treatment in pain reduction. These results held at six-month follow-up.
3. Cognitive behavioral treatment, including biofeedback, was more helpful in pain relief than symptom monitoring, although results didn't hold at eighteen-month follow-up.[108]

Reading more about the mind-body connection also can help jumpstart your program. These books provide an excellent starting point:

Moyers, B. (1993). *Healing and the Mind.* New York: Doubleday.

Goleman, D., & Gurin, J. (eds.). (1993). *Mind Body Medicine: How to Use Your Mind For Better Health.* Yonkers, NY: Consumer Reports Books.

Kabat-Zinn, Jon. (1990). *Full Catastrophe Living: Using the Wisdom of Your Body and Mind to Face Stress, Pain, and Illness.* New York: Dell Publishing.

Pennebaker, J. W. (1990). *Opening Up: The Healing Power of Confiding in Others.* New York: William Morrow and Company.

Zeidner, M., & Endler, N. S. (eds.). (1996). *Handbook of Coping: Theory, Research, Applications.* New York: Wiley.

Ornish, D. (1998). *Love and Survival.* New York: Harper Collins.

Pert, C. (1997). *Molecules of Emotion.* New York: Scribner.

Chapter 8

RELATIONSHIPS AND SEXUALITY

"Love conquers all: and let us too surrender to love."

—*Virgil*

Being in relationships is a basic part of being human—so much so, that we often take them completely for granted. Whether we're single or married, work at home or at an outside job, are highly social or more inwardly focused, we all depend on others to help us make sense of our lives, share companionship and laughter, and give and receive much-needed love and support during times of struggle.

Relationships have cycles and a rhythm of their own, ups and downs brought on by events in our own lives or those of others. These events can be internal (such as coping with depression, or dealing with the onset of RA), or external (job changes, moving, childbirth, loss of a loved one). These stressors affect many aspects of our day-to-day lives, including the way we interact with others—and, often, the way others interact with us. We might become irritable, for instance, or seem to suddenly look at the world through new eyes and emerge with a whole different set of priorities—and this can cause reactions in others. As you may have discovered already, the onset of RA can be just such a life event.

With the changes you may experience as a result of living with RA, your work, social life, activities, moods, and even your sexuality may at some point be affected—and, it goes without saying, many of your important relationships are likely to be affected as a result.

Relationships are a balancing act at the best of times, and this becomes more apparent when RA enters the mix. When the disease is taking a toll on your health—during a bad flare, for instance—you need to pay more attention to you, and less to those around you. Of course, we all need to nurture special relationships, and don't want to feel as though we're letting people down. If you're a parent or caregiver, or you've spent a lot of your life "doing" for others, it can feel like torture to have to pull back in this way—yet necessary for your own health and ultimately for those who rely upon you.

Similarly, how many times have you carried through with social engagements when you really didn't feel well enough? No doubt you were thinking of friends and family, not wanting to disappoint them, hurt their feelings, or make them angry. Do you ever lash out angrily at intimate friends and family because they just don't seem to understand how you feel? Or, do you keep that anger to yourself, letting it fester and add to your tension and pain? Do you ever feel like you want to throttle a loved one for offering you well meaning advice—or, worse, pitying you?

These are the kinds of relationship challenges people with RA and other chronic conditions sometimes face. Like anyone else, they value friends and family, but sometimes the effort that goes into maintaining those relationships is exhausting—it's a "can't live with 'em, can't live without 'em" situation.

On the positive side, major life challenges such as RA can cause us to open up more to others. For instance, you may find that sharing your feelings, or allowing others to help in ways that feel good to you, can deepen your intimacy. As a result of letting people get closer to you in this way, your relationships may actually become deeper and more satisfying.

Learning how to build strong, mutually supportive relationships brings enormous rewards for anyone who ventures to work at it—not just those who have RA. And the key, not surprisingly, is communication. In this chapter, we'll look at what people with RA, health professionals, and researchers have learned about how the disease affects relationships, then discuss some "how to's" of building and maintaining strong, supportive ones. We'll help you understand what your partner, if you have one, is going through as you face this disease together, and offer practical tips and support for maintaining a fulfilling sexual life. The chapter ends with a stand-alone message to partners of people who have RA.

RELATIONSHIPS

We all have days when everything goes right and all's well with the world. But introduce the slightest experience that could be described as negative, and our good mood can be gone in a blink. Not only that, we may not be able to shake off the negative feeling for some time. Research studies have shown that the negative effect on the psyche of any interaction that could be termed negative is *greater* than the *positive* effect of an interaction that's viewed as positive—both in the general population and with people who have a chronic illness.

With RA, you may from time to time experience a new sort of negative

interaction with others. There is evidence to suggest that people react negatively to someone who is ill or in pain, because it challenges a belief they
may hold that life is somehow fair. Perhaps unconsciously, they are reminded—and become fearful—that this could happen to *them*. Researchers have noted this pattern occurs with friends and family of people
with chronic illnesses and disability, as well as with casual acquaintances—
and even one-time meetings with strangers.

With the people closest to you, such as your partner or family members,
you may be affected by their genuine concern and worry about your health
but also by any resentment or anger they may be experiencing as a result of
any increased workload and changes in lifestyle or activities they've experienced since the onset of your RA.

Support

In a recent study, people with RA reported feeling most supported when
they are able to express feelings and concerns, when they receive hope and
encouragement, and when they are given *asked-for* information and advice.
They expressed most satisfaction when getting emotional support from a
spouse or partner, and more tangible support—such as advice on medications and pain management tips—from health professionals. Although
people can, when asked, break "support" down into a list of specific activities or behaviors, they also speak of "feeling supported in general" in a category by itself. In other words, the more supportive someone *feels* their
partner is overall—regardless of all the supportive activities they may be
undertaking—the less psychological distress the person suffers.

Under unhelpful support (it may seem odd to talk about "support" as
"unhelpful," but the people whose behavior was discussed thought they were
being supportive) several actions were described: minimizing the severity of
the illness; forcing cheerfulness; avoiding the person with RA; avoiding discussion of the illness; and being overly solicitous or pitying. Lack of emotional support from a spouse, ineffective help from health professionals, and
unwanted or unsolicited advice from friends were cited as unhelpful.

These findings confirm what other research has shown: There is sometimes a misunderstanding on the part of a friend or relative about what
constitutes "support," and when, how, and by whom it should be given.

It is clear to see what an important role communication plays in strong,
healthy, supportive relationships. If your partner and friends have to guess
what it means to support you, relationship breakdown and frustration—
for both parties—may result.

Communication

Even though we spend much of every day communicating in some way
with other people, most of us still find it hard from time to time. At work,

at home, and even in bed, clear, honest communication is absolutely essential to overcoming the challenges posed by RA. Learning to recognize and speak our whole truth in a way that others can really hear, and respond to favorably, is one of life's most difficult challenges. And hearing, respecting, and responding appropriately to another person's whole truth can be just as challenging.

The good news is that the effort involved in honing these skills is well worth it. Your relationship will benefit—whether it's with a colleague, romantic partner, close friend, or other significant person in your life—and your psychological health will be optimized.

Although many of these tips are intended for use in intimate relationships (such as the people we live with), many of the principles can apply to friendships and work relationships as well.

Try the following:

- Make an "I" statement rather than a "You" statement. For instance, you might tell your partner, "I feel helpless when you offer assistance without my asking for it," instead of "You are inconsiderate and don't care about me or you wouldn't keep stepping in and doing things for me." The formula is actually quite simple: Instead of a sentence like "You make me feel like [this] when you [do this]," try saying "I feel like [this] when [this] happens." That way you're not accusing anyone of anything, and you're leaving the door open to talk about your feelings—and the other person's feelings as well.
- Stay in the moment; don't use words that blow things up, such as "never" and "always."
- Make a statement instead of asking a question. For instance, you might say to a colleague, "I find it difficult to manage my priorities and do my job well when you give me such short notice about deadlines," instead of "Why don't you tell me these things a little sooner?"
- Be quick to be accountable when you have need to be, and be as fully accountable as you can. "You're right. I wasn't able to do that and I know it was important to you. I'm sorry. I'll get it done first thing tomorrow morning. Will that work for you?"
- Be generous with apologies. Saying "I'm sorry" does not necessarily mean that you would do it differently if you could do it over again, or that you are wrong. It can simply mean that you recognize that someone is hurt or suffering, and you are sorry about whatever way that you being you has contributed to that (even if you are perfectly innocent and the other person was surprisingly triggered because of things from their past which have nothing to do with you).

- Be liberal with thank yous and general gratitude. Notice when someone is working hard in the conversation with you, is being accountable for something that is hard for them to acknowledge, or is using their compassionate inner strength to see things from your perspective instead of reacting from their own. Let them know you see their generosity and are grateful for it.
- Avoid using words that mitigate the strength of what you mean. It can make you a traitor to your own feelings and also confuse what you are saying. For example, saying "it bugs me" when it actually infuriates you is unclear communication and does not give the other person accurate information to use when deciding whether or not to do the offending thing again. Using mitigating words also can prevent you from conveying positive feelings. For instance, your spouse's statement, "I can't believe my luck in having you as a partner" followed by your response of "I *sometimes/ kind of/sort* of feel the same way," loses an opportunity for deeper intimacy, if in fact what you feel is the same way.

Special tips to help when you're angry:

- With the individuals closest to you, you may wish to negotiate in advance some rules of arguing that enable both of you to feel safe and comfortable. For example, some people feel raising their voice (yelling) is essential to "getting it all out," while this is threatening and feels unsafe to others. Some people need to walk away and come back when they are feeling rational and as if they have it all figured out—but their partner ends up feeling frustrated and abandoned during the interim. So set time aside when you are feeling loving toward one another, and use it to make an agreement about how you'll behave when you're angry. Each person should have an opportunity to share what works best for them, what frightens them, what makes them even angrier, and so on. It helps to have this agreement in writing if there are several issues you as a team have decided on. Then, stick to the agreement the next time you have an argument. You are grown-up enough, have enough control, and love each other enough to honor such an agreement, even when you are feeling your wildest.
- You may want to take an agreed-on timeout for fifteen to twenty minutes before talking to each other when fury strikes. During the timeout, do something to relax or distract yourself, to help your compassionate self resurface. It may again help to agree to this timeout principle even before the argument strikes; it can

help when there is a difference of opinion between you about whether walking out in the middle of an argument is okay.

- Be careful not to call the other person names or label them (for example, "you are a control freak") and if they call you a name, let them know it is not acceptable.
- Try not to purposely say things that will harm or incite the other person
- Of course, no violence is acceptable (which includes throwing objects, hitting things, slamming doors).
- Take turns listening. When you talk, keep it about yourself; the point of talking is to reveal yourself and be vulnerable to your partner. The listening person's job is to not to react, but to be extremely curious about their partner's inner experience.
- Try "mirroring"—you say something to your significant other, they repeat what they heard, and you tell them if they missed anything or misunderstood you in any way. Mirroring will develop your active listening skills, helping you understand what someone is feeling and thinking as opposed to just saying. Plus, your partner will feel like you've really heard and understood them.

YOUR LIFE PARTNER

Pairing up can be good for your health. On average, married people (whether legal or common-law) live longer than single people (those who have never married, or are divorced, separated, or widowed). Although you may link that finding to the positive effects of companionship in general, that doesn't explain it fully: married people also have longer life expectancies than single people who live with friends or other family members.

Marriage also can be bad for your health—if your relationship is troubled, for instance. Research shows that people who are unhappily married experience poorer health than their happy counterparts, including less effective immune system functioning. People who are separated or divorced—in other words, who have experienced marital tension—tend to be less healthy than those who are happily married and even those who have never been married or are widowed.

We've been discussing the general population. Now let's look at what the research says about how RA changes the picture. These general findings are confirmed: If you're comfortable in your marriage, your stress level will be low and you'll suffer less depression about your RA—and so will your partner. There's even evidence to suggest your disability will increase more slowly than that of people who are not married or are unhappily married. That's in the best of situations, of course, and the best of situations don't just happen—partners bring them into existence and nurture them constantly.

As difficult as RA is for you, it's important to realize that it also has profound impacts on your partner. He or she is possibly taking on more responsibilities at home, providing care and support, perhaps dealing with a reduced social life, experiencing the effects of any depression or anxiety you may be experiencing, and of course feeling upset because you are suffering. There is a strong relationship between your level of distress and your partner's level of distress. Perhaps because emotions are so powerful, and your connection with your partner is an emotional connection, the psychological changes you may be going through have a more significant impact on your partner than the physical aspects of your disease.

Research into other chronic diseases has shown that a partner of someone with the disease experiences depression, anxiety, poor immune function, stress, psychosomatic symptoms, and less than optimal functioning at work. These results seem to hold true for partners of people who have RA.

If this all sounds terribly negative, as if your relationship is doomed—it's not. Accepting that RA can negatively affect your partner—which in turn will affect your relationship, and you, means you may work even harder to overcome the potential difficulties.

One of the ways you can do this is by encouraging your partner to seek psychological or emotional support outside the relationship, which has been shown to be extremely helpful. If your partner is male, you may have to encourage it strongly: Men (more so than women) generally rely on a spousal relationship as their primary social tie, which means they may not have preexisting social supports, and will be less likely to ask for help from other people.

Communication with those closest to you can be really tough—in part because there's so much at stake if it goes wrong. And when you have to talk about emotionally charged issues it gets even tougher. When communicating with your partner, try to use the principles we discussed earlier. If your partner is up for it, consider using the following questions as starting points for in-depth, intimate conversations or mirroring exercises to do together.

Ask the Person with RA

- What "support" do you find most helpful and least helpful?

Ask the Partner

- When is supporting me the most difficult for you (this can be internal factors, such as when you're tired; situational factors, such as when the children are being demanding; or things about the partner with RA that make it difficult to support them at different times)?
- Do you feel appreciated? What makes you feel appreciated?
- Are there ways that you would like me to support or give to you that you have been reluctant to ask?

Ask Both of You

- What are the losses you have endured as a result of the RA (things in your relationship, personally, in your social life, and even for your dreams and hopes for the future)? It's good to acknowledge them or consider whether there is a way to reclaim some of them in your life.
- Are you satisfied with the amount and quality of your lovemaking? What brings you the most pleasure? What do you wish there was more of? Less of? Are you having any feelings about sex that you haven't expressed—guilt, anger, disappointment? Is there something new you would like to try (that perhaps you feel bashful about)?
- Acknowledge each other: The strength, courage, and compassion each of you has demonstrated has no doubt been of heroic quality. Take time to tell your partner about the wonderful things you have noticed in her/him. Include the big things and the little things that your partner might not have realized you noticed.
- Acknowledge your relationship: As a team, you have been through a tumultuous sea. Acknowledge the qualities in your relationship together that have carried you through these sometimes difficult and sometimes wonderful times.
- Include the whole family: Where possible, and as appropriate developmentally, include children or other involved family members in these discussions. It is helpful for everyone to have a chance to share their feelings about the impact of the disease on their lives, to have their pain and their strengths acknowledged, and to be told how much they are appreciated and loved.

For more tips, see Kate Lorig and James Fries, *The Arthritis Helpbook* (specifically the chapter on feelings and communication); or consult the myriad of self-help books in most shops, including *The Dance of Anger* by Harriet Learner. For support in communicating, don't hesitate to find a therapist who specializes in couple's counseling, or if only one of you wishes to get support, find yourself a good therapist or begin sharing your thoughts and feelings with a friend (see Chapter 3 for more information on this).

SEXUALITY

Is it possible to have a healthy and satisfying sexual life despite living with a painful, tiring, and sometimes debilitating disease? Yes. However, as with everything else we've discussed, it does take a bit of work and planning.

The majority of people with RA who took part in research studies a number of years ago considered sexual problems to be within a physician's scope of practice, and indicated they would be most comfortable receiving advice on this topic from their doctor. Unfortunately, the subject of sex is still relatively taboo in our society, even among doctors and other health professionals, who rarely raise the topic with patients—perhaps wary of their patients' potential discomfort with such a discussion. In other words, each party is waiting for the other to raise the topic.

Will RA Affect your Sex Life? The Research Says Yes, and No

It's easy to imagine how fatigue, depression, pain, decreased ability of joints to move—all symptoms of RA to varying degrees—could affect a person's sex life, including their desire for lovemaking.

But the data vary wildly in terms of satisfaction with sex after the onset of RA. Although some research into RA and other chronic illnesses has shown a detrimental effect on sexual desire, arousal, and orgasm, a significant number of people in some studies report no change in their sex lives as a result of the RA. For some, sexual fulfillment may even increase as a result of the deeper relationship that a couple can develop through enhanced communication.

All that's conclusive is that the percentage of people with RA reporting dissatisfaction with their sex lives is higher than in people who don't have a chronic illness.

If There Are Problems, What's Causing Them?

If you are experiencing loss of sexual desire, or difficulty with the physical acts of lovemaking, consider the following four potential causes.

PHYSIOLOGICAL CAUSES

Problems such as pain, fatigue, and limited range of motion are likely the primary causes of sexual difficulties in people with RA. For obvious reasons, pain and fatigue often can cause dramatic reductions in an individual's sexual desire (who wants to make love when they have a splitting headache all over their body?). And, of course, limited range of motion can cause practical problems with the physical act of lovemaking. For example, hip and knee joints tend to be particularly troublesome, making it challenging for many people to assume comfortable positions. Also, vaginal dryness due to Sjögren's syndrome (see Chapter 2) can make intercourse painful—if this is the case for you, try using a lubricant jelly, available at any pharmacy.

PSYCHOLOGICAL CAUSES

Libido-decreasing effects of RA include depression, anxiety, fear, concern over body image, and lowered self-esteem. Many people choose to be single and are happy with the freedom and autonomy of this lifestyle; however, some people have trouble after a diagnosis of RA finding the energy, motivation, or self-esteem to seek a partner. For some people, RA brings about unwelcome changes in their view of themselves as a sexual being.

MEDICATION-INDUCED CAUSES

Decreased libido (sexual desire) is a side effect of some medications used to treat RA. Research has shown that corticosteroids such as prednisone, muscle relaxants, narcotics, and drugs to treat depression may decrease libido or cause impotence (inability to sustain an erection).

RELATIONSHIP-RELATED CAUSES

This is a wide category, including marital unhappiness, a partner's fear of hurting their mate, a partner's disinterest, or embarrassment over difficulties with sex as a result of the disease. Either party may suffer guilt (a woman with RA may just not be well enough to make love; her partner may feel awful for even thinking about sex when she is so ill) or resentment (someone with RA may feel pressured to have sex even though they don't feel well enough; their partner may feel angry that every aspect of their life seems to be affected by the disease).

It's interesting to note how women with RA rank relationship-related sexual problems compared to men with RA. For women, pain is the biggest problem, followed closely by "problems with a partner" (including her partner being afraid of hurting her during sex, a partner's disinterest, relationship problems, her feeling responsible for his sexual satisfaction, problems with sexual roles). "Lack of partner" and "fatigue" were next in priority. For men, by contrast, pain was the biggest problem, but then came lack of interest in sex, then fatigue—partner problems were not even mentioned. If you're a woman with RA, you'll be able to see how important a role communication plays in a fulfilling sex life. All the issues raised under "problems with a partner" can be addressed and eased considerably by talking them through. You may find the tips on communication described earlier in this chapter helpful in this regard.

What to Do

The sexual difficulties that arise for some people with RA can be considerable. But if a fulfilling sexual life is important to you, it's worth working through those challenges. Here are a few tips.

PREPARING FOR LOVEMAKING

Try preparing for sex as you would for other types of physical exertion:

- apply moist warm heat to joints or other areas of the body that may be painful during sex
- take a warm bath or shower—with your partner, if that's something you would both enjoy
- do some range-of-motion exercises to warm up your joints
- take painkillers thirty minutes beforehand (so that their peak of action will coincide with your lovemaking time)
- put on some romantic music to help your body relax and release tension (and therefore, release pain as well)

DURING LOVEMAKING

- when laying on your back, have pillows under your hips to aid pelvic extension
- if kneeling, place pillows under your knees to support painful or contracted joints
- if you have severely limited movement in your joints, or if repetitious movement causes discomfort, try a water bed, which facilitates movement
- engage in sexual pleasures that can be accomplished with comfortable positions, such as oral sex, mutual masturbation, "talking" sex, intimate touching, or using sexual aids
- for intercourse, the positions illustrated in Figures 8.1 to 8.5 will help to ease the strain on stiff and/or painful joints (especially hips, knees, and spine), and do not require as much range-of-motion as other positions

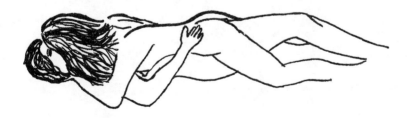

Figure 8.1. In this position, there is no prolonged pressure on the man's joints.

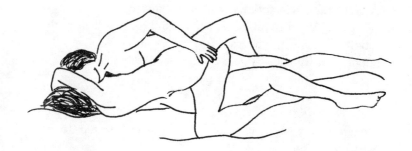

Figure 8.2. In this position, neither partner has prolonged pressure on their joints.

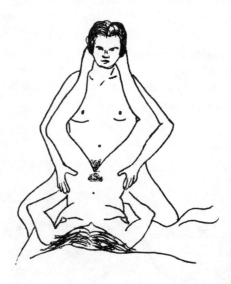

Figure 8.3. A woman who is unable to straighten her hips might use this position.

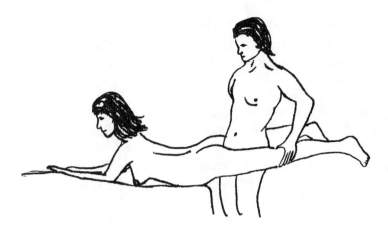

Figure 8.4: This rear entry position might be useful for a woman who is unable to bend her hips or knees.

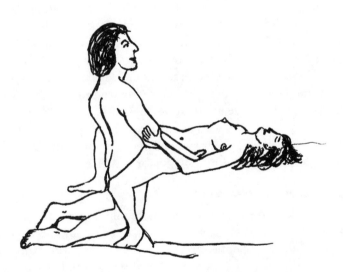

Figure 8.5: A woman in this position does not have prolonged pressure on any of her joints. A woman who is unable to bend her hips or straighten her knees might find this position comfortable.

Illustrations by John Marsala, adapted with permission from Buckwalter, K. C., Wernimont, T., and Buckwalter, J. A. "Musculo-skeletal conditions and sexuality II." *Sexuality and Disability*, 5 (4): 195–207, 1982.

PROFESSIONAL HELP AND RESOURCES

A good therapist (for example, a skilled psychologist or specialized sex therapist) can help you work wonders for your sexual life. Consider seeing one if you need to:

- help you and your partner talk about sex
- reassure your partner they will not harm you by making love with you
- assist you and your partner change the way you think about your sex life, with the primary focus on intimacy rather than particular goal-oriented sexual acts
- recommendations for books, tapes, workshops, or other resources—here are a few to get you started:

   The Passionate Marriage, by David Schnarch, published by W. W. Norton

   The Passionate Marriage workshops, at www.passionatemarriage.com

   Tantra: The Art of Conscious Loving, by Charles and Caroline Muir, published by Mercury House

   Good Vibrations, is an international mail order and publishing company with two retail stores. In business for more than twenty years, Good Vibrations promotes itself as a "clean, well-lighted place for women and men to buy and learn about sexual products." They believe that "accurate sex information encourages better communication about sex, which in turn promotes health and happiness." For more information on workshops and products (books, movies, and sexual aids that can be ordered discreetly through the mail) go to www.goodvibes.com or, in the United States, call toll-free 1-800-289-8423 for a catalog.

MEDICAL/SURGICAL TREATMENT

Although not done for sexual problems alone, hip surgery can considerably decrease pain and increase range of motion. In one study, the surgery alleviated hip-related sexual difficulty in 95 percent of the participants. Thirty-five percent of the participants still reported sexual difficulty due to other factors, however.

Whether you're a sexually active single person or have a life partner, take comfort from the fact that you are not alone with your questions and frustrations about sex. Few people, regardless of their health status, report sexual relationships they are completely happy with, so throwing RA into the mix is sure to complicate things. A formidable challenge, yes, but like most challenges, one that you can overcome with persistence and a plan.

A Message for Spouses and Partners of People with RA

This message is based on the relationship, nursing, and professional counseli experience of contributor Sharon Demeter, M.A., M.S., R.N., C.N.M., whose partner lives with a chronic illness.

Take Care of *You*

Being the partner of someone with a chronic illness has unique challenges and can be very difficult. For the sake of enjoying the best quality of life available to you, being the best partner you can, and counterbalancing the physical and psychological health risks that your situation poses, it is important to prioritize taking good care of yourself.

This can be hard because the demands of life may already seem to take more time than you've got—so generating energy to even *think about* how to care for yourself may seem impossible. Or, perhaps you would feel guilty thinking about self-care when it is your spouse you believe you should be caring for. If that sounds familiar, consider this: The amount of time you spend being good to yourself (whatever that means to you) will pay off in a significant increase in the energy and willingness you have to take care of your spouse and the rest of your life.

Most people know deep down what makes them feel good; if they think about it, they can list the activities and pleasures that rejuvenate them and add to life's rewards. Eating well and exercising are obvious places to begin, and we heartily encourage you to do both. But it's also important to take care of your needs for pleasure and relaxation. If you're feeling too guilty or stressed to do this, here's a place to begin: Make a list of things you would really love to do. Try not to censor yourself with thoughts such as "I could never find time to" or "She/he would be mad if I ..." or "That's a silly thing to want to do." List activities that you would find fun, relaxing, exciting, or rewarding. They can be small (such as an hour-long shower or an uninterrupted video marathon) or big (a whole weekend at home without chores; a skiing trip). Just jot down whatever comes to mind that would be enjoyable for you.

Next, decide to do one of the things on your list. Hopefully, after one rejuvenating experience, the benefits of enjoying yourself will be persuasive enough to encourage you to make it a habit.

It's also important that you not stop doing the things you love. If going for a bike ride makes you feel good but you haven't had the time lately, make an effort to carve out the time. Also, be sure to get emotional support for yourself—talk to friends or family about what you are going through, join a support group or a men's group, or see a therapist. Remember that you are not betraying your partner by acknowledging negative feelings about their illness or the demands it places on you. Quite the reverse: having a third party bear witness to any resentment or anger you may feel will help you get if off your chest, and you'll become less likely to unintentionally express these feelings in harmful, indirect ways toward your partner.

Here are a few more self-care ideas: get a massage, get away for a long weekend, embark on a long-term plan to do something you've always wanted (such as hiking in Nepal, becoming a fabulous cook, buying a Harley, or pursing a different career).

Finally, be sure to get practical support when you need it. The ups and downs of RA, particularly during the early stages when the disease is uncontrolled, can demand so much time and energy that it leaves you both exhausted. During times like this, you might arrange to have a family member to pick up your groceries; a couple of friends each bring over a casserole once a month on an ongoing basis; a cleaning service take care of heavy housework, or a neighborhood teen clean up the yard, walk the dog, or play with the kids while you take a nap. People are usually only too happy to help: they just need to be asked.

It's important to reassure yourself that it's okay to let some things fall by the wayside or be done by others, if it means you can keep up with the high priorities of maintaining your health, supporting your spouse, and maintaining a healthy, fulfilling relationship during a time of tremendous strain for both of you.

Give Good Support

Research clearly shows that what spouses imagine to be helpful is not necessarily perceived as being so by their partner. This may not seem to apply to you, but it's worth having a conversation with your spouse about it. Consider asking them what they find particularly helpful, what they don't find helpful, and what they would like more or less of. If you discover discrepancies, conflict and bad feelings might ensue—but know that these will be short-lived, and the conversation will amount to a more positive relationship in the end.

After all, this friction in the relationship is understandable. You may discover that you have been providing an "unhelpful" type of support for a long time without realizing your partner's perception of it. Or your partner receiving the "support" may feel unseen or misunderstood; unacknowledged because they have tried to express their needs clearly and do not feel you have responded; guilty acknowledging that certain things don't feel supportive (believing they should just feel grateful for all that you are doing for them); or hurt or angry because you don't meet their needs the way they would like. You may feel some anger that you have been "wasting your time" doing things for your spouse that weren't helpful, or feel hurt that the ways of giving support that feel good to you aren't received as gifts of loving support by your loved one. Any other reactions can ensue. The important thing is to talk to each other, listen to each other, forgive each other, and move into a deeper level of understanding, cooperation, and intimacy. And, ultimately, of course, make sure what you're doing for your partner with RA is what that person wants and needs.

Forgive Yourself for Not Being Superhuman

The role of the partner can, in some ways, be as challenging as that of the person with chronic illness. It is very normal to feel resentful that this has happened to you, furious (at God, the doctors, your children, your spouse), sorry for yourself, depressed, frustrated, unappreciated, overworked, and utterly exhausted.

Accept that your feelings are common and understandable. Feel them, and find a way to talk about them. Ideally you can share them with your spouse, but sometimes it can help to express them to friends or a therapist. It's also important to give meaning to your feelings and listen to what they are telling you. Do you need a break? Are there certain things that you are doing that are soul-killing and must find a way to change?

Don't feel guilty for not being an unwavering angel of generosity: What you are doing is hard. Self-punitive judgments confuse things, and shut down the rest of the feelings, which usually means the feelings don't end up getting shared. What does not get said will often find other ways of being expressed (in outbursts, illness, accidents, nonsupportive actions toward our spouse, forgetting, and confusion). So, avoid telling yourself "I shouldn't be feeling this." It would actually be more unusual *not* to feel these things at least some of the time. When these feelings are chronic, persistent, and intrusive, it is a sign that they have not been adequately listened to. Get help from a professional or a friend who is supportive, nonjudgmental, and a good listener.

Feeling Alone

If you met your partner before he or she developed RA, then all of the ways RA has changed your spouse may leave you feeling like you're alone—like you've lost your best friend. The amount of your partner's energy now being used to manage pain and symptoms is energy that is not available to you and the life you once had together.

Rheumatoid arthritis can be divisive: You can empathize with but not truly understand your spouse's experience living with this disease. Your partner's world has been significantly and perhaps irrevocably altered in a way that you will not ever fully comprehend. The world you both once shared may be becoming only a painful memory to your partner. The roles you may have once taken for granted in your spouse—sexual partner, social partner, recreation partner, active co-parent, or co–wage earner—may be diminished or even seem like they are gone for good. So, it can leave you feeling like RA has come between you and left you alone in the world.

There may be some painful truth to be acknowledged if you have lost valued and significant aspects of your partner for which you yearn. It's important that you and your spouse get these feelings out in the open (in a loving, safe way, such as through use of the communication exercises described earlier in this chapter).

Fear and Uncertainty

Like your spouse who lives with RA, you probably have tremendous fear and uncertainty about what the disease means to your lives: What course will it take? How can you help manage your lover's pain? How will your family be managed? How will you cope financially? These questions may be accompanied by feelings of helplessness, hopelessness, and loss of control. If that describes yours, you might consider reading Chapter 7, which explains many of these feelings and offers practical advice and tips for getting through them.

Blaming Yourself, Blaming Your Partner

Some people blame themselves for somehow bringing on the RA in their spouse (they caused their partner stress, didn't appreciate them, etc.). This is wrong. Other people blame the partner with RA (they have unresolved psychological issues that they are unwilling to work on, so now they're sick and torturing both of us with the illness, and so on). This is also wrong. There's no research to support these views, even though for decades the researchers were intent on trying to find evidence that would support either blaming the "victim" or their family. It's not uncommon in the face of uncertainty, and feelings of being overwhelmed to start blaming, but refuse to do so. Choose healthier alternatives, such as expressing your feelings and taking care of yourself. It will be better for everyone.

Finding Meaning

What good has come out of your partner's RA? Have there been any lessons? A realization of deeper love or commitment? A new surrender to the ways of the universe? Deeper faith?

It is just as important to acknowledge the positive outcomes as it is to acknowledge the losses and suffering the disease has brought on. Research has shown that those who find meaning in ostensible misfortune fare better: They are healthier, happier, have better relationships, and suffer less distress. So, if it is possible for you to imagine this disease in a larger context that makes it meaningful to you, then do so. You might wish to get support in this regard from your religious, spiritual, philosophical, or social network to the extent that you find it helpful.

Chapter 9

WORK, FAMILY, AND LEISURE

"Problems are only opportunities in work clothes."

—*Henry J. Kaiser*

Many people who develop RA become suddenly aware of how they once took for granted their ability to perform everyday activities. From the smallest of tasks such as opening a door or brushing one's teeth to the larger responsibilities of running the house, providing for the family, and holding down a job, the "activities of daily living," as occupational therapists refer to them, can take on a new significance.

If you're struggling with activities that once seemed basic, you're not alone. Painful joints, restricted mobility, and fatigue can cause many people with RA to leave the paid labor force or cut down significantly on the number of hours they work outside the home, participate less in social and recreational activities, and to some degree become dependent on others for assistance with certain tasks.

However difficult some physical activities may be, take heart: It *is* possible to limit the negative impact of the disease on your day-to-day life and continue to work, care for your family, and pursue most of the activities you enjoy. An occupational therapist or OT (whose job it is to show you how to handle the demands of everyday life and get things done with a minimum of pain, stress, and fatigue) can help identify solutions to many of the activities that create problems as well as help you find innovative ways to continue doing the things you love.

It's a good idea to make an appointment with an OT experienced with RA, who may even be able to visit your home to suggest adaptations to work areas, furniture, or other home modifications if needed. To find an OT who understands RA, ask for recommendations from your rheumatologist or national arthritis organization (Arthritis Care in the United Kingdom does not give referrals, but The Arthritis Foundation in the United States and The Arthritis Society in Canada do). See Chapter 13 for contact information. Of course, there's a lot you can do by yourself to overcome the challenges involved in taking on the day. And it all comes down to *optimizing your environment and use of energy*—step "O" in the PLAN TO WIN.

Let's start by learning how to look at an activity that causes you problems. Then we'll discuss three ways of approaching solutions. We'll also look at some ideas for adapting your self-care, leisure, recreation, and work activities.

WHAT'S THE PROBLEM?

Identifying the problem is the most important step toward finding a solution. It may sound obvious, but it's easier said than done. For instance, to identify the problem as a general activity such as "making dinner" or "playing cards" or "gardening" doesn't get at the root of the problem, or pinpoint what's really causing the trouble. What is it about making dinner that's difficult? Are the pots too heavy? Are the cupboard handles too hard to grasp? Are you simply flat-out fatigued by the time dinner is on the table?

Potential solutions for problem activities are plenty. Drug stores and health specialty shops are full of new and improved gadgets and gizmos for making various activities easier. Many of these devices are great, but it is essential to make sure you know what you need before you buy—if indeed you have to buy anything at all. How? By getting as close as you can to the "why" of the problem. That will help you decide whether to adapt the task itself or your approach to it, get help with certain parts of it, do it at a different time of day, or in some cases, even decide against doing it (or in favor of delegation).

Incidentally, this chapter is for you even if you aren't experiencing difficulty with specific tasks. Making activities as easy as possible on your joints is smart disease management, and will help ensure you keep your joints functioning.

CREATING SOLUTIONS

Once you've identified the problem, apply the following three solution-oriented principles:

- adapting the task
- protecting your joints
- making optimal use of your energy

Often all three principles can be applied to one activity, and will work together to allow you the greatest possible level of independence in doing that activity.

1. Adapting the Task

USING AIDS

Once you know the core of a problem, one of the first questions to ask is yourself is: How could I adapt this task to make it (finish this sentence with the result you want to avoid, such as "less fatiguing," "less painful," or "less stressful on my joints")?

It's natural for people to want to resist adapting activities, especially with tools that in some way look "medical." Many people feel that using a long-handled reaching stick, a cane, or a raised seat of any kind is giving in to their disease, somehow being beaten by it. Although the feeling is understandable, nothing could be further from the truth. Adapting activities will make them easier, allow you to have more pleasure in your life, and, more important, it will lessen RA's hold on you, because you're not weakening your joints or otherwise stressing them. Think of adapting activities as preventive and proactive.

There is a wide variety of devices on the market these days that reduce the amount of effort needed to do a job. Increasingly, these devices are losing that medical or institutional look and feel, and they're now sold in most pharmacies, department stores and specialty kitchen shops—not just medical supply stores.

Some of these devices, such as long-handled shoehorns, sock aids, and reaching sticks, will extend your reach so you don't have to strain. Others will allow you to apply more force to a task by using leverage—tap turners, L-shaped knives, and lever doorknobs fall into this category. Look for tools that reduce the chance of your hands slipping off a surface—for instance, jar openers—and those with fat handles, which will minimize joint stress.

DOING THE TASK IN A DIFFERENT WAY

Of course, you can also adapt activities by simply doing them differently. Using the principle of getting the most traction, use a wet cloth or a rubber sham to help you get the top off a bottle. Or, to avoid having to grasp a refrigerator or cupboard door handle with your fingers, attach a loop of string, rope or decorative cloth to the handle, and leave it there. You'll be able to put your forearm through the loop and pull the door open using the strength of your whole arm.

Another example of adapting an activity is to do it in stages. Instead of cleaning the whole workshop at one go, spread out the individual tasks—

organizing the tools, sweeping the floor, wiping the windows—over one or several days.

2. Protecting Your Joints

Another important problem-solving question to ask yourself is, "How can I protect my joints while doing this activity?"

Occupational therapists define "joint protection" as the use of any technique that reduces external stress on disease-affected joints. That means performing activities a certain way to protect your joints, as well as using adaptive equipment or specific tools designed to make an activity easier to perform.

The following information for the most part deals with joint protection during activities, but there is much you can do at rest as well.

PROTECTING JOINTS WHILE AT REST

Splinting

To protect your joints while you're resting, splinting of your wrists or fingers may be required. A splint is a type of orthotic, usually made from hard plastic, that immobilizes the joint and allows it to have maximum rest. Keeping a joint at rest is especially important if it is inflamed. (Even if there are days when joint rest is needed, taking them through their full range of motion once daily is best—see Chapter 5 for more on this).

Apart from wearing splints (you'll need to be fitted for these by an occupational therapist), you can protect specific joints by using pillows for support. When you're sitting, for instance, keep a small pillow or rolled towel in the small of your back, or use an Obus Forme back support. And a small towel in your pillowcase (rolled into the shape of a small log and snuggled into the small of your neck) will protect your neck while you sleep on your back. Custom-made shoe orthotics are another important joint protection option for many people with RA: These fit in your shoes and keep your foot in position, minimizing pain and joint damage. As always, consult an orthotic or splint maker who is familiar with RA. Ask an occupational therapist or other health professional for more resting joint protection techniques based on your body's particular needs.

PROTECTING JOINTS DURING ACTIVITY

The golden rules of joint protection during activity

- Avoid repetitive movements (typing on a keyboard, operating certain machinery, and so on) and static postures (sitting or standing still for long periods of time). These will put strain on the joints you're using to do the activity or maintain the position. If you must do repetitive movements, it's a good idea to move or change positions often to avoid stiffness, and stretch and relax often. Ask

a physiotherapist to recommend specific stretches for the task you
are doing.

- Use large, strong joints and muscles instead of small ones for carrying, pushing, and pulling objects. For instance, put groceries
  into a bag you can carry on your shoulder rather than with your
  hand. Or use a collapsible, wheeled grocery pull cart. Instead of
  using your finger to push the nozzle of a spray can, use the palm
  of your hand. Whenever possible, use your whole body instead of
  just one part (slide the garbage cans rather than carrying them, or
  better still, get the ones on wheels). You'll reduce joint stress and
  prevent joint pain.
- Distribute any load over as large an area as possible: Use two
  hands instead of one to lift your coffee cup, carry a plate, or get
  clothes from the closet. Use the palm of your hand to hold an object such as a saucer or a photograph, rather than holding it by its
  edges with your fingers, if pinching movements are painful.
- Extend your reach to avoid bending. Here's where good adaptive
  equipment such as sock aids, long-handled shoehorns, and garden hose nozzle extenders, available through arthritis organizations and medical supply stores, comes in handy.
- Use what occupational therapists call, "good body mechanics":
  using your muscles and joints efficiently in order to reduce stress,
  pain, and fatigue. Practice good posture: when you're standing,
  imagine a string connecting your ankle, knee, hip, shoulders, and
  ears and pulling up through the top of your head. Don't lock your
  knees (keep them very slightly bent); keep your shoulders back
  and your pelvis tucked. As you sit, keep your hips, knees and ankles at a ninety-degree angle. Over long periods of time, varying
  positions frequently is adviseable.
- To stand up from a sitting position, get as close to the edge of
  your chair as possible. Place one foot ahead of the other, keeping
  the forward knee and foot aligned (the other foot remains behind). Lean forward until your hips start to come off the chair,
  and then push up with your arms. Using a padded cushion on any
  seat will increase your height off the ground, making it easier to
  stand up.
- Good body mechanics is also vital when you're lifting objects
  (avoid lifting heavy things if at all possible): keep the object close
  to your body; keep your knees bent; keep your back straight.
- Maintain muscle strength and joint range of motion through exercise and gentle stretching (see Chapter 5 for practical information and tips on therapeutic and recreational exercise).
  Remember, protecting your joints doesn't mean not using them at

all. It means being wise about how you use them, and not pushing them beyond what they can do.

3. MAKING OPTIMAL USE OF YOUR ENERGY

The final of our three problem-solving questions to ask is, "How can I make the best use of my energy?"

On days when you wake up with lots of energy, feeling better than you have for ages, it's tempting to take advantage of that get-up-and-go feeling, accomplishing as many things as possible while you can. Go ahead and enjoy this energy surge, but try not to overdo strain on your joints or burn yourself out. After all, even the healthiest people burn out quickly if they don't conserve energy. When you have RA, the burnout can be worse: You can end up exhausted, in pain, and depressed for days afterward.

Planning

The key to an effective plan is looking ahead to enable you to optimize your use of your energy, just as any effective business manager would do. Many health care professionals recommend planning activities a week in advance. It's a good idea to use a diary or journal, and write down everything you want to accomplish on each day of the week—including leisure activities and rest times—and then prioritize the items. Schedule the most strenuous activities for when your energy level is generally the highest. Alternate the heavy and light activities, and schedule in rests after the most rigorous. If you're inclined to work through breaks when you don't feel tired, set a timer and obey its signal.

You're much more likely to be realistic about what you can accomplish if you view the entire week ahead at a glance. And once you've been through a week or two and can look back and see how much you can do, you'll be even more realistic about the weeks ahead.

Of course, your week's plan is never written in stone. In fact, it's better not to expect to get everything on your list done. The idea is simply to plan and prioritize, so you get through the things you must and most want to do with an appropriate amount of rest in between. If you have a particularly good week, you get more done than if you have an off week. Be flexible—if someone invites you sailing and you feel great and the sun is shining, go for it! Or if you get through only two things on your list and you're exhausted, take it easy and rest.

Another benefit of using a diary to plan for your week ahead is that you can keep notes each day on what worked and what didn't work. Perhaps you'll jot down a reminder not to clean the kitchen *and* paint it in the same week again, or maybe you need to rest after different activities from the ones you originally thought. Your diary is a good place to record suggestions on how to adapt activities as well—a kind of "idea file." Once you start to realize how much easier activities can be, you will be thinking of, and hearing about, new approaches all the time. You might not be able to follow up on all of them at once, but you can collect them for future action.

Conserving Energy By Doing Tasks Differently

As well as conserving energy through scheduling activities for certain times, think about how you can save your strength by doing tasks differently. Sliding objects instead of lifting them, using large, strong joints and muscles instead of small ones—all the principles mentioned in the above sections will also work to maximize the use of your energy.

Whatever activities are involved in your day, apply the concepts of adapting activities, protecting your joints, and wisely using your energy. Here are a few ideas to get you started along those lines, under the general headings of self-care, productive work, and leisure activities. Think of these ideas as a starting point: your unique solutions will depend on your occupation, your hobbies, your RA disease activity, and your approach to activities in general.

SELF CARE

Hygiene

The bathroom can be a frustrating place for anyone with pain and restricted mobility—brushing or flossing your teeth, combing your hair, and scrubbing your back, for example, require the kind of movements that can be excruciating if you have swollen or sore joints. Bathrooms are also potentially dangerous sites, given the slippery surface of bathtubs and wet floors.

Fortunately, there are some very useful alterations you can make to your bathroom that will help ensure your safety and maintain your independence.

Grab bars by the toilet and in the bath make a world of difference for anyone who needs extra support or help getting up from a sitting position. Also helpful is a raised toilet seat (or a toilet installed on a platform, for those who dislike the institutional look of a raised seat). The idea here is to raise the seat just high enough to make it easy to stand up.

If you find it difficult to stand in the shower, or are afraid of falling, try sitting on a bath bench or stool and using a long-handled spray attachment to give yourself a shower. Some benches have an opening so you can wash the genital area.

If you find it hard to perform the motions of brushing your teeth, try an electric toothbrush.

Once you start looking into "bathroom aids" you'll find things you never thought of: decorative toothpaste squeezers, flossing aids, nonslip tweezers—the list is endless.

- use a nonslip mat in the tub to decrease the chance of falling and increase your confidence
- use a bath mitt with soap sewn into it to save a bar of soap flying out of your hands.
- if possible, have lever taps installed—these are much easier to turn on and off than round knobs.
- a fluffy terry cloth robe works wonderfully as a towel
- use liquid dish and bath soap, shampoo, and conditioner in pump jars—and use your palm, rather than a finger or thumb, to press the pump handle
- for hairbrushes and other implements, look for big, nonslip handles with an extended reach, or cover the handle with pipe insulation (this magic solution can be used on any handle to increase the size of its grip).

Besides adapting your environment and the tools you use, think about how else you could conserve your energy or make the tasks easier. For instance, if you've always wanted to get a short haircut, maybe now would be an opportune time to enjoy a short style that requires little maintenance. Also, try brushing your teeth and doing your hair after your shower: Your muscles will have loosened up from the hot water and movement, and your joints will probably have a greater range of motion.

Dressing

When choosing your wardrobe, it's a good idea to invest in clothes that you feel great in *and* can get into and out of with a minimum of pain and frustration in the event that you experience a bad flare. Some practical clothing tips to consider:

- try to buy clothes you feel dazzling in, that *don't* have tricky buttons, belt buckles, suspenders, or zippers—you also might consider replacing small zipper pulls with larger decorative ones available at sewing stores
- if you have a flare that causes sore arms or shoulders, choose loose-fitting clothes with larger neck and armholes—they're the most comfortable, and the easiest to get on and off
- use a long-handled shoehorn to help you slip into your shoes easily, without bending or crouching
- wear slip-on shoes such as loafers as often as possible; avoid shoes

that require lacing up (many fashionable running shoes now have Velcro closures)
- if you tend to wear button-up shirts or pants, get an inexpensive button hooker—it's a metal loop that goes through the button hole, grabs the button, and pulls it through
- use the very handy device sometimes referred to as a "sock aid" that will eliminate the need for stretching to put on and pull up your socks
- choose elastic waistbands over zippers where possible
- for women who experience difficulty pulling on panty hose, consider wearing pant suits on days when hands are painful
- sit down to get dressed
- give yourself lots of time to get dressed so you don't get frustrated

WORK: AT HOME AND ON THE JOB

Cleaning

If it's possible—and we know this is a tall order for some people—consider lowering your cleaning standards. Isn't your health is more important than a dust-free laundry room? And spending time with your family more important than an always spotless kitchen? Unless the sight of unmade beds really bothers you, do you need to do more than simply straighten the covers every morning? Do you have to wash the car every weekend?

Also, try to make cleanups a family responsibility. As a group, decide at the beginning of each week which chores need to be accomplished, and divide them up. Even small children can take on a small task, and it will get them used to helping around the house as they grow older.

It's a good idea not to take on more than one major cleaning job a day. And try to allow yourself lots of time. Take frequent breaks, listen to music—whatever will help make the job as easy and pleasant as possible.

Some more cleaning tips:

- use a wheeled cart to take your cleaning supplies from room to room, or store them as close as possible to where you'll be working
- sit down to sort and fold freshly laundered clothes
- eliminate ironing time: buy permanent press—or, if you can afford it, send items that need ironing to a laundry.
- use long-handled tools when possible: dusters, reachers, toilet brushes
- use spray cleaners to break down stains and caked-on debris, and minimize the need for scrubbing
- use a dusting mitt

The best tip of all: If you can make room in your household budget, hire a housecleaning service twice a year for a thorough spring and fall cleaning, and get by with maintenance the rest of the time.

Cooking

If you love cooking, it's well worth getting an occupational therapist to visit your home and suggest adaptations to your kitchen. Things such as cabinet height, counter height, pullout shelves, and arthritis-friendly storage of various utensils and food make a world of difference, and an OT will think about things you may not consider. Some adaptations are expensive, but if your time in the kitchen is a creative outlet for you, seriously consider making them, perhaps one at a time as you can afford it.

There also are inexpensive tools you can buy, and simple new approaches to kitchen tasks that will help immensely.

Consider these:

- sit, rather than stand, to peel vegetables
- invest in a chair on wheels—one high enough so you're not reaching up to the counter
- check out the amazing number of adapted kitchen tools on the market: jar openers, reachers, large-handled, lightweight coffee mugs, light dishes, adapted vegetable peelers, and more
- plan meals ahead, getting the family to help
- make double portions of everything and freeze half for another dinner
- use electric appliances rather than those that are hand-operated
- use disposable pans and plates occasionally, to minimize clean up and give yourself a break
- place a wet cloth under bowls to stop them from slipping while you mix
- ask a handyperson to hammer metal skewers up through the bottom of a cutting board so you can secure your vegetables while you chop
- organize your cupboards so the most often-used and heaviest items are within easy reach—for example, pots and pans are usually stored in low, hard to reach cupboards so consider relocating the ones used most often so that they are closest to waist height, to reduce the strain of retrieval
- use a sieve spoon to take food out of boiling water, rather than lifting a hot pan to the sink and draining it
- make simple meals and get the kids to help—there are some great recipe books on the market specifically for people who have limited mobility (try *The Essential Arthritis Cookbook*, by Sarah L.

Morgan, or *Help Yourself—Recipes and Resources from The Arthritis Foundation*)

- take advantage of having family and friends help in the kitchen by getting together and preparing several days' (or several families') meals at once
- use precut fresh vegetables (you can even buy ready-made salad at supermarkets these days, and the quality is generally very good)
- alternate tasks such as chopping and stirring to reduce stress on your hands
- storage considerations: lazy susans, pegboards and hooks
- develop a repertoire of one-pot meal recipes, for easier cleanup
- shop for grocery items at one store instead of three or four specialty shops, and be open to improvising if they don't have exactly the right fruit or vegetables for your planned meal
- ask about free grocery delivery
- keep your knives sharp
- if you're having company over, opt for a potluck meal
- if there are kitchen tasks you would always prefer to avoid (such as filling or emptying heavy pots of water), negotiate to have your spouse handle them on an ongoing basis, so that don't have to ask

Caring for Children

Although you may not feel like talking with your children about your RA, it's important to try to find a way to address it. An open, honest relationship with your family will help alleviate the anger, depression, and stress that can build up in children of any age, particularly when they don't understand things that are happening around them.

Research has shown what most people with RA know by experience: the disease can decrease one's ability to manage a household and nurture family members.[1] One study showed that families with a mother who lived with chronic pain had poor perceived family environments and experienced more depression and anxiety than other families.[2] The same is true of spouses of people who live with chronic illness—for in-depth discussion of issues and tips related to life partners, see Chapter 8.

By contrast, many parents who have a disability report that their children are well-adapted, mature, perceptive, and respectful of others' feelings.[3] No doubt these are the parents who have recognized the importance of talking with their children about the realities of their condition.

Your children need to understand your disease and how it affects you. And, strange as it may seem, they can develop that understanding at a very early age. They also need to be encouraged to talk about how your having RA affects them.

You will need to create a system of communication that works for your family—some way they can remain tuned in to your perhaps frequently changing energy and pain levels. Simply talking about how you're feeling at any given time might work, but some people find it irritating to constantly have to report on their condition or answer people's inquiries as to their health. Many people use something like a scale of one to ten, or a series of faces ranging from happy to anguished, to communicate to their children how they are feeling that day. If your kids understand your pain or fatigue is "about an eight" one day, they won't be requesting that their friends come over after school—and you won't feel guilty about saying 'no.' They may even pitch in a little more with the housework. If you're a one or two out of ten, the kids can look forward to a more cheerful and energetic you, and they'll respond accordingly.

The above-mentioned suggestions for dealing with housework and cooking—discussing the weekly chores as a family and who should do what—will help immensely. It helps to work as a team to create new ways of doing things, even leisure activities.

One thing you will have to work on yourself, however, is letting go of any guilt you may be experiencing over not being a perfect parent or a perfect partner. No one is. Everyone lives with some challenge, and yours happens to be RA. And besides, self-blame, guilt, and anger makes people feel tense, which adds to pain—and your goal is to *break* that pain cycle. So please be gentle on yourself.

Women with arthritis say that the most difficult aspects of baby and toddler care are breast-feeding, putting the little ones into a crib, playpen, or car seat, and dressing them. Adapted equipment such as that mentioned in the list below will help, but try as much as possible to schedule difficult activities so that family and friends can help. Perhaps you and your partner can bathe the baby at night (leaving the lifting to your partner), or a neighbor could help the baby into the car seat when you need to go out. You'll be amazed at how willing people are to help—especially when they know exactly what it is that you need.

Here are some more hints for caring for babies and toddlers:

- choose diapers depending on the challenges you face with your hands—disposables are great if you have shoulder trouble and find laundry difficult, but the little tabs can be too difficult to manage for some people with RA in their hands (you might wish to consider a diaper service that offers snap-on closures or big Velcro tabs in this case)
- choose clothes with Velcro closures rather than snaps (or have someone alter the clothes for you)
- wear wrist splints, which give good support for holding babies, and pick up baby using a scooping movement with your whole forearm, rather than just your hands.

- childproof the house as much as possible, so you're not rushing all over trying to prevent falls and breakages
- get one or two spoons with fat handles for feeding baby
- lift your child in stages to reduce stress on weak muscles—pick him up and hold him on the floor, then move to a sitting position in a chair, then stand
- slings or shoulder-mounted baby carriers (such as Snugli® or Baby Björn®) can help you pick baby up. For example, if you are lying down together, put baby in the Snugli® and then stand up, rather than bending over and picking up baby with your hands. But be careful, since these devices can be painful on shoulder, neck, and back joints if used for any length of time
- purchase or borrow a lightweight, easy-to-fold stroller
- add castor wheels with safety locks to baby's high chair
- get older children involved in caring for a baby brother or sister

For more helpful tips on caring for baby, see Chapter 11.

As your children get older, you will face different challenges. When they are school-age, it's helpful to form a network of people with kids the same age, and share responsibilities with other parents. For instance, they can take the kids tobogganing or whatever it may be that you find difficult, and you can do homework duty, take the kids to the library, or supervise them while they play.

One of the most beneficial things you can do, both for your kids and for you, is to lower your expectations of their behavior. They may grumble about taking on chores, but that's normal. They may occasionally make a mess of a chore—that's also normal. Encourage them to do it right next time rather than be cross at them for messing up this time, and make a concerted effort to notice them doing things right and give them lots of praise. They will be much more likely to keep pitching in, and will slowly develop a strong sense of the integral role they play within the family.

Shopping

With the growing popularity of shopping for groceries over the Internet and having them delivered, you may be able to eliminate this task altogether. However, you may not want to. Many people enjoy a daily or twice-weekly trip to the market to check out the freshest produce or get inspiration for an evening meal.

Here are a few ways to make shopping as easy as possible:

- use a trolley or a wheeled cart, rather than bags, to carry groceries
- go out to shop, but get the groceries or goods delivered—many stores offer this option, some without charge
- shop for small specialty items yourself, but ask others (family or

neighbors) to buy canned goods, sacks of flour, and so on when
they buy their own
- take several short shopping trips through the week instead of one
long one that might tire you out
- if you drive, take advantage of the parking for people with disabilities right near entrances (ensure that you have a permit if one is
required where you live)
- when you're carrying groceries, hold them close to your body or
use a shoulder bag, backpack, or big pockets

Employment

If no obvious accommodations need to be made to your workplace, your
schedule, or your position, you may decide not to tell people you have RA at
all. Or perhaps you'll begin with telling one or two trusted colleagues, as a
way of testing the water and getting practice. It's up to you, but do bear in
mind that people who don't know you have RA won't know you may need
support from time to time. And if at times you need to take frequent breaks
or delegate certain tasks, resentment may build if people don't know the
reason and support you.

That said, never before has there been so much awareness on the part
of employers about the importance of accommodating employees who
have physical challenges or disabilities. Motivated by the need to keep
valuable employees, and also by the desire to adhere to laws, many companies are ensuring their environments are barrier-free, comfortable
places to work.

That's not to say you won't have to do any education of your own in the
workplace, however. For one thing, RA is often an invisible disease—you
can be in the greatest of pain but the only thing that may give it away is your
facial expression. For another thing, awareness of RA and its effects is still
quite low. When you're ready, you may need to educate your co-workers
and employer about the disease, if you haven't already done so.

If you have a job and are experiencing difficulties fulfilling its responsibilities, or if you're looking for a job, it's worth making an appointment with
a vocational rehabilitation counselor or a social worker. Such professionals
can assist with a number of employment-related matters. They can help you
discover what type of job would be a good fit for your needs and abilities,
advise you of retraining opportunities should you wish to change career, or
make suggestions on how to adapt a current situation to better accommodate your health needs. They also can advise you of your legal rights as an
employee with a disability or as one who needs to be accommodated.

In the United States, workers are protected by the Americans with Disabilities Act, which bans discrimination against people with disabilities in
hiring and employment. In Canada, the Canadian Human Rights Act obli-

gates an employer to accommodate an employee with a disability "short of undue hardship."

In other words, it may be too much to expect an employer to completely remodel expensive machinery so that you can continue to use it. A more realistic expectation is that your employer would discuss with you new opportunities in the same workplace. Other reasonable accommodations an employer must make include adjusting your schedule or working hours, allowing you to switch from full-time to part-time work, arranging for you to trade tasks with a coworker, changing the height of working surfaces, and so on.

If you belong to a union, its agreement may have a "disability clause," and the union may support you in pressing your employer to make changes to your work situation.

Some people with RA don't want to raise the subject of arthritis at work for fear of losing their job. It's unfortunate, but it is a reality for some people. Before you raise the issue of arthritis and possible workplace changes with your employer, decide how far you want to go down that path. If they refuse to cooperate, or lay you off, do you want to file a complaint against them and the company, or even press charges? Think about what your life would be like if you were successful, and the company was forced to accommodate you. If you work in a big organization and rarely see your employer, you may be perfectly satisfied with the outcome. But if your employer or coworkers resent you for fighting your case and you're constantly reminded of it, you may end up thinking you've "won the battle but lost the war."

If possible, keep the relations between you and your employer amicable. Present your case as an opportunity for your employer to help you work to your best potential, rather than as a problem they must fix. Before you meet with your employer, prepare a list of suggestions for how the challenges could be met. They will appreciate your having done some homework, and will perhaps be more open to listening to the possibilities. Enlist the help of social workers, vocational rehabilitation counselors, occupational therapists, and other members of your health care team—they will help get your employer on your side, and remind them they are lucky to have you.

Here are some tips for ensuring your workplace situation is geared for maximum satisfaction:

- be honest with yourself about what it takes to get your job done, and your ability to do it
- make your workspace as efficient as possible: arrange items to minimize lifting, reaching, and carrying
- pace yourself—alternate between light tasks and heavy ones
- sit to work whenever possible, in an easily adjustable chair
- use a footrest

- if you're working at a desk, make sure your chair, computer, telephone equipment and other high-use items are positioned for maximum ease of use and so as not to cause you unnecessary strain—an occupational therapist or specially trained ergonomist can help here
- take advantage of modified tools such as pens with fat handles (or add inexpensive foam pipe insulation—available at hardware stores—to regular pens)
- ask your employer to install pull-out shelves
- work shifts that correspond to your high energy times
- consider job sharing if that is an option, to reduce your total working hours or days
- trade joint-stressing tasks with a coworker or negotiate them out of your job description
- ensure correct chair and desk height (again, an ergonomist or occupational therapist can help)
- every half hour—or any time you feel joints stiffening or muscles tightening—take these areas through their full range of motion two to three times.
- give your eyes a break by looking away from the computer screen every once in a while (your eyes will benefit from having to refocus)

If you've tried all the options and ultimately your current job isn't working out for you, consider changing your job—even working independently from home, if you have the self-discipline and a marketable skill.

Start by listing your talents, skills, and strengths—you will be amazed how many you have. That list forms the beginning of your new career plan. If there is a job you're interested in doing, list its responsibilities, and note by each one how it will affect your health, if at all. The popular book, *What Color is Your Parachute* by Richard Bolles (Ten Speed Press), can help lead you through this process.

If you feel overwhelmed by the thought of looking for a new job or changing careers entirely, try to focus on the knowledge that somewhere out there is the perfect situation for you—one that will keep you feeling productive and connected with the world, but that doesn't leave you with no energy for anything else. As mentioned, a vocational rehabilitation worker or social worker is the person to call on for job-related concerns, whether you need support and encouragement, or practical assistance finding resources or retraining opportunities.

Leisure

Leisure—the time you spend away from work-related or productive duties—is vitally important to your optimal health. When active, RA can dull one's interest in leisure activities, primarily because it affects one's ability to perform them. Even something as simple as reading is a problem when it hurts to hold a book.

If you talk with occupational therapists, other people with RA, or visit specialty stores, you'll probably find that there are solutions to many of your leisure-related problems. Can't hold a book without it hurting? Place it on a pillow, or invest in a manufactured bookrest.

There are card holders for the bridge player, and adapted needles for the knitting enthusiast. If needlepoint becomes impossible, because of the tight grasp it requires and the stiff position of the neck, think of taking up macramé. Or continue to do needlework, but for limited periods at a time or when you're feeling good. Consider the psychological benefits of doing something you love; do they outweigh any negative physical effects of the activity?

Here are three examples of leisure activities—gardening, travel, and entertaining—and some hints on how to make the most of them.

GARDENING

Start by assessing your situation: How much you can bend and lift? Which tasks cause you pain or stress your joints? How long you can work before you get tired? Then, design a garden—or a gardening routine—to suit your unique situation. You might consider joining a garden club for help and ideas in getting set up (your local garden store or the library should have a list of clubs).

More ideas:

- use long, fat-handled garden tools
- take frequent breaks—use a kitchen timer to remind yourself if necessary
- alternate tasks to use different muscle groups
- be realistic—don't grow a jungle; even one lovingly tended box can be a rewarding gardening venture
- learn about raised-bed gardening—basically, planter boxes on stands a few feet above the ground—which all but eliminates the need to bend
- make sure you have lots of room on pathways
- ensure there are no slippery surfaces in your garden
- look into watering options—water is heavy: you can get two-handled watering cans, or a hose with a series of stopped-up holes down its length (which eliminates the need to move the hose around the garden—just lay it out once, turn it on, and unstop the holes nearest to the plants that need watering)
- serious gardeners who can afford this option might consider installing an underground sprinkler system

- for the heavier tasks, see if someone from a service or kids club can help
- do a little every day, rather than too much one day and nothing for two weeks
- keep your tools sharp and well-oiled
- use ground covers, mulch, or rock in place of lawn, so you're not having to cut it frequently, and plant flowering evergreen shrubs and trees that don't require much maintenance or cleanup
- design your garden so there are several pleasant rest areas
- drink lots of water as you work
- learn about container gardening, or hanging-basket gardening, if you're working with an apartment balcony or in a small space
- sit on a small stool rather than kneeling
- pad the handles of tools with foam pipe insulation to enlarge the grip
- carry tools in an apron with a pocket
- store tools, seeds, and supplies as close to where you're working as possible

TRAVEL

If you love to travel, these days there is no reason to be limited by your RA. People who work in the travel industry—agents, airline staff, tourism office workers—go to great lengths to ensure the needs of people with physical challenges are met.

Your best bet is to get a good travel agent and make them aware of your needs. They will be able to find you accessible hotels, ensure you have transport, if necessary, in an airport, and so on.

Some more travel tips:

- choose the right trip—you may have always dreamed of hiking down the Grand Canyon, but will you enjoy it?—and ensure that you train appropriately to meet the physical demands of your adventure
- be careful not to schedule all your free time with sightseeing tours; plan for rest and recovery time—and ensure your travel companions know you'll need to do so
- stay in hotels close to a taxi stand or public transportation
- stay in hotels equipped with grab bars in the shower, raised toilet seats if necessary, and so on
- check if the hotel has amenities such as irons and hair dryers—you'll have less to carry that way
- ask for a room with close access to the hotel's amenities

- invest in lightweight, wheeled luggage
- stay in hotels near the areas or attractions you wish to visit
- if you're on a driving holiday, stop every hour to stretch for a few minutes
- in a car, plane, bus, or train, do range of motion exercises frequently
- pack lightly and do laundry more frequently
- wear and pack comfortable clothing
- if you need it, consider requesting a wheelchair for sightseeing tours or in the airport
- ask porters to carry your luggage
- when traveling by air, inform airline staff ahead of time as to your needs (an aisle seat, help to the washroom, a wheelchair to the baggage area, etc.)
- do as much as possible ahead of time so that you'll spend less time waiting when you get there; reserve not only airplane seats, but also sightseeing tours and restaurant tables; take advantage of the express checkout option available at many hotels and car rental agencies
- if you rent a car, get one with power steering, brakes, windows, and locks
- for your own car, check out some helpful adaptations such as seat belt cushions, tilted steering wheels, and the warm and grippable steering wheel covers such as those made from sheepskin
- when you book your flight, inquire about the distance you'll need to travel between check-in and your departure gate. Allow extra time between flights to travel this distance, or arrange for alternative transportation (such as a wheelchair or a ride on one of the chauffeured carts provided as a courtesy by many airports)
- make rest an enjoyable part of your holiday; relax and enjoy parks, hotel pools, movies, reading, leisurely meals, and coffee breaks

ENTERTAINING AND SOCIAL EVENTS

While it may be too difficult to invite fifteen people over for a five-course dinner, having some friends in for a potluck supper can be just as much fun.

As usual, planning is key. Plan the evening well in advance, making a list of things that need to be done. Spread the tasks over several days, getting help with any cleaning you may need to do. Keep it a casual occasion—you might even use paper plates and plastic cutlery. Ask each guest to bring one dish, and lay it out buffet style. Everyone will be happy to pitch in—the important thing is being together.

For more formal affairs, ask a teenager to help out in the kitchen and with serving the meal—then treat them to a movie the following week.

Asking for Help

No chapter on "living day-to-day" would be complete without a section on communicating with others about the help you require (and, of course, the help you don't require).

Some people find it very hard to ask for assistance, perhaps because it means admitting they can't do everything themselves. If that's you, then first of all remind yourself than no one—regardless of how healthy they are—can do everything alone.

If you've devised a communications system with your family as discussed earlier, you've taken the first step. For instance, if your children and spouse understand you're at "eight" on the pain scale, they'll understand you will be requesting more from them throughout the day, and it shouldn't be too uncomfortable for you.

Practice being forthright in your ask for help, for instance saying "Could you please load and unload the dishwasher this morning?" rather than "I need some help with housework." People feel most helpful fulfilling a specific request.

Once your family and friends come to realize that you'll ask for help when you need it, they won't offer help when you don't want it, which can be disempowering as well as extremely irritating to people with RA. Practice declining offers of help gracefully when you're well enough to do things on your own, indicating that help "some other time" would be welcome.

As for strangers, you'll find them quite happy to help you, particularly if you're specific about what you need. Many people with RA have no visible symptoms at all, so if you wait by the grocery shelf hoping someone will get you down a can of tomatoes, you'll likely stand there a long time unless you ask for help.

Optimizing your environment and use of energy will take you a long way toward being able to accomplish the things you want to in life. Remember, there is no such thing as "normal." Everyone has unique strengths, weaknesses, needs, and abilities. The most important thing is to decide what you want to do, then find a way of doing it—with help if need be. As a wise person once said, no one is ever given a wish without the possibility of making it come true.

Chapter 10

SURGERY

"Wherever the art of medicine is loved, there is also love of humanity."

—*Hippocrates*

Since surgery is far from being a certainty for people with RA, it seemed appropriate to reserve this chapter in the PLAN TO WIN as one of the last. In fact, if your disease is well controlled by the other components of your treatment plan (medication, exercise, physical and occupational therapy, mind-body work, among others), you may never need surgery to help manage the consequences of RA. However, for those with long-standing moderate to severe disease dealing with the hardship of daily pain or loss of joint use and disability in their life, surgery could be a saving grace.

The goals of surgery in RA are threefold: to reduce pain, to prevent joint damage, and to improve one's ability to function day to day.

Coming to grips with needing surgery may actually be the most difficult part of the procedure for some people. For others, the commitment to months of postsurgical rehabilitation might seem daunting. Whichever the case, making the decision to have surgery requires careful consideration.

As with the other aspects of your PLAN TO WIN, having reliable information to refer to, and experienced, trusted health care team members to call on, is critical. Working as a team, you will get the education and emotional support you need to make the best decision possible and enjoy optimal results.

TIMING IS EVERYTHING

When RA pain is inadequately controlled by medications, exercise, physical and occupational therapy, among others, and causes a person to be unable

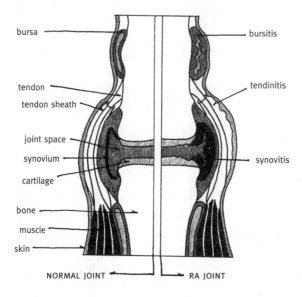

Fig. 10.1. Normal joint on the left and RA joint on the right. The synovium is a thin lining that makes the fluid that is present in small amounts in a normal joint. The fluid nourishes the joint and lubricates it. In RA, the inflammation of the lining thickens it, more fluid is made, and the joint swells as a result. The inflamed lining can damage the cartilage and nearby bone by releasing inflammatory substances and by direct attack. The lining of tendons is similar to the lining of the joint. It can become inflamed in RA. Finally, a bursa is literally a small sac that normally protects a tendon or joint. A bursa also has a lining that can become inflamed, resulting in extra fluid production and swelling.

to do even basic things like standing, walking, holding a fork, and hair-brushing, surgery can be an excellent option.

Determining when or whether you need surgery is the first step. To get the best results from surgery with the fewest complications, the time to be evaluated for surgery is *before* you need it. Delaying surgery can actually lead to deformity, contractures (shortening of tendons or overlying skin), and muscle atrophy (shrinking muscle), all of which prevent chances of good recovery,[1] and may compromise your long-term results from surgery.

For example, a knee might suffer unnecessary bone erosion and destruction if acute and persistent synovitis (inflammation of the joint synovium; see Figure 10.1) is present in the joint for a lengthy period of time. A synovectomy (removal of the inflamed tissue), when performed at the right time under the right circumstances, can delay or prevent damage, giving the knee—and its owner—a new lease on life.

The issue of timing becomes more complicated if multiple joint surgeries are needed. If an individual requires both wrist and knee surgery, it may be best to have the wrist surgery first, given the person will need the use of it to manage crutches or a cane when knee surgery follows. Conversely, if surgery on both knees is needed, it might be best to have the surgeries performed simultaneously; otherwise, the total recovery period may be prolonged, or the person may favor the treated knee over the untreated knee, causing an imbalance in use and, possibly, instability when moving around.

Another factor to consider when timing surgery is whether and when postsurgery support is available to you at home or at work: Having family or friends by your side to help with housework, meal preparation, and personal grooming will make the first few days and weeks following surgery a lot easier to handle. If you're employed, find out what type of short- or long-term disability insurance you may have and whether the services of physical and occupational therapists are included in the coverage.

Your rheumatologist and orthopedic surgeon are in the best position to determine when you may need surgery, based on your disease severity, joint status, medication regime, and physical and nutritional health. You, however, play an integral role in bringing factors such as lifestyle, mental and emotional wellness, and support network, into the decision-making process.

BENEFIT VERSUS RISK

Deciding whether or not to have surgery is all about weighing the benefits versus the risks—just like you do for other aspects of your treatment plan. Only then will you and your health care team feel completely comfortable with the end decision.

Benefits

The two key benefits of surgery are pain relief and improved movement and use. Both offer a tremendous positive impact on a person's quality of life.

Another benefit of surgery is improved appearance, particularly for severely damaged joints. Although rheumatologists and surgeons will rarely, if ever, recommend surgery for cosmetic reasons alone (when weighed against risks of surgery), improvement in the appearance of a joint postsurgery offers a valuable psychological benefit.

Risks

Along with the benefits surgery can deliver, come potential risks: Some can be "predicted," and others cannot. With careful and thorough planning, you and your health care team may be able to minimize the risks, especially those health factors that can actually predict poorer surgical results.

Things that may jeopardize good surgical results:

having a heart or lung condition: these and other serious health concerns should be under control prior to having surgery; otherwise,
the stress and strain of surgery may pose too great a health risk

poor general health: being physically fit and in good general health
not only makes one feel better, but preserving strength and range
of motion can help speed the postsurgery recovery process (one
reason for not delaying surgery is that severe pain and disability
often leads a person to get out of shape)

poor diet and nutritional status: maintaining a good diet can improve the body's ability to heal after surgery and can help minimize the risk of infection and other complications

being overweight: carrying excess weight on the body means greater
pressure on all the joints during recovery, and is associated with
slower return to good function

**unwillingness or inability to follow an appropriate postsurgery re-
habilitation plan**: being willing and able to commit to a postsurgery rehabilitation plan is critical to gaining back good
function. The person having surgery will need help handling their
usual tasks around the home and at work. Family members,
friends, and coworkers must understand that they will have to
"pitch in" and help as your function may be limited for some time
after surgery; and you must think long-term—extra effort in the
recovery period can mean many years of optimal function and
range-of-motion

RISKS DURING AND AFTER SURGERY

Sometimes, no matter how carefully the plan is laid, risk still exists. Below
are some of the complications that may arise during or after surgery—
some are serious:

- extensive blood loss
- nerve and blood vessel injury or damage
- postsurgical infection or delayed infection (possibly weeks or
  months after the operation)
- chance of blood clots
- loosening or rapid wearing out of artificial joint replacements

The three most commonly occurring complications after surgery are infection, blood clots, and loosening of artificial joint replacements.

Compared to people with osteoarthritis, individuals with RA who undergo joint arthroplasty surgery (see page 200) get infections afterward
more frequently,[2] although chances of getting an infection have been re-

duced over the years due to improved surgical procedures and the use of antibiotics at the time of surgery. Corticosteroid and methotrexate use and the immunologic process of RA itself could contribute to developing an infection. Signs of infection in the replaced joint include pain, warmth, or redness of the overlying skin.

Blood clots occur most often in hip and knee replacement surgery. In hip replacement surgery, it may be because of the person's anatomic position (lying flat) during the procedure; in knee replacement surgery, it may be because blood flow in the leg is restricted during the procedure. Whatever the reason, individuals undergoing hip or knee replacement surgery should be given blood thinning medications for a period of time after surgery to reduce the chance of blood clots.

The major cause of artificial joint replacement failure is because the artificial joint becomes loose in the bone into which it is glued. Pain is the key symptom of a loosening joint. If persistent, even mild pain is felt, the person should see their surgeon to have the joint X-rayed to determine the best course of action for repair.

It is important to remember that the risks of complications are rare and they should not deter you from seeking surgical advice. Your surgeon can clarify how these risks pertain to your case and discuss concerns with you.

QUESTIONS TO ASK YOUR RHEUMATOLOGIST AND SURGEON

To help you assess the benefits and risks surgery may hold for you, gather information from the two players on your health care team who know your disease and your prospects for successful surgery best—your rheumatologist and surgeon. Below is a comprehensive list of questions you should ask before making your decision.[3] Record answers in your health journal so that you can review the information in the comfort of your home and with the help of family or friends, if needed. If appointment time is limited, leave the list of questions behind and ask your physician to follow-up with you after the appointment on the telephone or in writing.

Sample list of questions:

- Are there other treatment options besides surgery effective at treating my problem? What are they?
- What are the chances nonsurgical treatment will be effective?
- Can you explain the operation to me and the expected results in "nonmedical" language I can understand?
- Do you hold board certification to perform this surgery?
- How many times have you performed the recommended surgery on someone with RA?

- What risks are involved in the surgery? What is the chance of these risks occurring?
- What are the risks if I delay or don't have the surgery?
- Do you have written materials, pictures, or videotapes on this surgery that I may borrow?
- Would you give me the name of another person with RA whom you've performed this surgery on to talk to me about it?
- Will I be admitted to a hospital, or can the surgery be performed on an outpatient basis?
- How long does the surgical procedure take?
- Are blood transfusions necessary? Can I donate my own blood in advance?
- What level of improvement can I expect after the surgery?
- Will I need surgery again?
- Will my GP be involved with my care in hospital?
- Do I need to stop my RA medications before or after surgery? If so, what type of medication will be used to control my disease during that time? Are there risks associated with this medication?
- Are there exercises I could do before or after the surgery that would help speed my recovery?
- How many days or weeks will I be in hospital?
- Will I be in a lot of pain following the surgery? Will the pain last long? Will I be given medication to help control the pain? What kind? Will I become addicted to it? Will I need to take medications after I leave the hospital?
- How soon can I get out of bed after surgery?
- How soon does physiotherapy begin after surgery? How long does each physiotherapy session last? Will I receive physiotherapy at home, in a clinic, or in a rehabilitation hospital or nursing home?
- Will physiotherapy be covered by my medical insurance? (This question should be asked of your insurer prior to surgery. Some insurance companies may stipulate that these services be preauthorized.)
- How limited will my daily activities be when I return home from the hospital?
- How often will I need to see you for postsurgery follow-up appointments? Are they included in the cost of surgery? If not, does my insurance cover the cost of these follow-up visits? (This question should be asked of your insurer prior to surgery. Some insurance companies may stipulate that these services must be preauthorized.)

The following questions relate specifically to joint replacement surgery (arthroplasty):

- Will I be able to feel an artificial joint in my body?
- How can I prepare for having joint replacement surgery?
- Can I have multiple joints replaced at once? Should I?
- How many times can I have the same joint replaced?
- Are there recreational exercises I will not be able to do with an artificial joint replacement?
- What are the latest advances in joint replacement research?

BEFORE AND AFTER SURGERY

Before

Much of the mental and physical preparation before surgery is like that of a runner getting ready for a 10K race. Well before the race, the runner takes special care to include a nutritionally balanced diet as part of their training plan. They also study the race course beforehand, figuring out where the challenging sections are and developing a strategy to perform well through those sections. The person with RA having surgery should do the same.

Eating nutrient-rich foods prior to surgery and during the first full year after surgery helps the healing process.[4] Pay particular attention to getting enough vitamin C before and after surgery, as it is essential to the body's tissue repair process. Because smoking interferes with the body's absorption of nutrients and is known to pose myriad other health risks, quitting before surgery is strongly advised.

In addition, knowing the surgical "game plan" can take the mystery away and possibly make you feel more confident and in control. Below is an example of a step-by-step timeline for knee replacement surgery, a frequently replaced joint in RA. Your surgeon and your hospital will likely have a protocol (way of doing things) similar to the following:

- Before being admitted to a hospital for surgery (usually several days prior), an internal medicine specialist or your family doctor will assess your overall health to confirm you are fit enough to undergo anesthesia (the process of putting and keeping you asleep during surgery). Provide the internist with a written list of all medications (and dosages) you are taking at present, particularly if you are taking aspirin or aspirin-like medications or prednisone (or other form of cortisone) on a regular basis.
- If you wish to, you can go to the hospital once or twice, three to five weeks prior to surgery, to donate your own blood for use during surgery (called "autotransfusion").
- A week before surgery, you will: have your urine and blood tested; an electrocardiogram (a heart test) administered; a chest X-ray

taken; and visit with the anesthetist (the doctor in charge of putting you to sleep during surgery). Also, the surgeon or one of their staff may give you information about the surgical procedure itself, and about what to expect immediately following the surgery.

- A day before surgery, call the hospital to confirm what time you need to arrive and the time of the surgery.
- On the day of the surgery, you will be admitted to the hospital and assigned a room. About an hour before the surgery, you will be taken to the operating room for premedication; the knee being operated on will be scrubbed with iodine and then shaved. You will then be given medications by intravenous (into the vein) to put you to sleep. Then you may be given general anesthesia by a breathing tube into your throat to keep you asleep. At that point your surgery will be performed. The procedure usually takes about three hours. After the surgery, you will be taken into the recovery room, or, if either the anesthetist or the internist feels it's necessary, to the intensive care unit.
- The day following surgery, you can get out of bed and sit in a chair, and possibly put full weight on your knee if there were no surgical complications.
- Two to three days after surgery, you will probably be able to stand and take steps with the help of a physiotherapist.
- Three to five days after surgery, you may either be transferred from hospital to a rehabilitation center or go home, depending on your individual needs, medical coverage, and the type of arthritis program offered in your community. In either case, you will begin a light physiotherapy program designed to reestablish range-of-motion in the knee.
- Two to four weeks after surgery, you should see the surgeon again for a progress checkup, and continue with light physiotherapy.
- Shortly after surgery, you should begin a comprehensive post-surgery rehabilitation program, preferably, with a physiotherapist experienced with joint replacement rehabilitation in RA. You may be able to resume driving and certain other daily activities depending on your rehabilitation progress. Your rehabilitation program should be individualized to meet your specific needs.
- You will see your surgeon for checkups approximately three months and one year after the surgery.

TYPES OF RA SURGERY

Described below are a number of different surgical techniques used in RA to prevent, delay, or correct damage caused by the disease.

Arthroscopy

Think of an arthroscopy as the orthopedic surgeon's "window" to the joint. Through an arthroscope (a thin tube with a light on the end that transmits a picture on a closed-circuit TV) inserted into the joint, the surgeon can assess the type and extent of the damage. A synovectomy and tenosynovectomy (see below), cartilage repair, joint smoothing, tissue biopsy, and loose tissue removal can all be performed during an arthroscopy.

Arthroscopic surgery has two main advantages over other surgical procedures: very little anesthesia is required, and the person can usually recover from the surgery and start walking much sooner because not much cutting is involved.

Synovectomy

The primary goal of a synovectomy is to prevent cartilage and bone destruction by removing diseased synovial tissue (see Figure 10.1 on page 192) lining the ends of bones that meet to form a joint. Removing diseased synovium can be part of a procedure to help realign and stabilize a joint. This procedure is usually performed arthroscopically.

A radiation synovectomy is one in which a radioactive substance—such as Ytrium—is injected. The synovial cells in the joint absorb the Ytrium, permanently damaging them. Ytrium loses its radioactivity very quickly. This type of synovectomy is more likely to be used in those who are not, or no longer, thinking about having children. Because this type of surgery is performed through a needle rather by cutting through skin and underlying tissue and muscle, only twenty-four to forty-eight hours of bed rest is needed after surgery before one is able to resume full activity.

Whether a synovectomy or radiation synovectomy is performed, the synovium may grow back in several years time if the RA is not controlled. As a result, the procedure may need to be repeated.

Tenosynovectomy

Tendon sheaths are much like a joint lining. They can become swollen and limit the normal movement of a tendon, thus limiting the movement of a joint. Also, the inflamed tissue can damage the tendon itself. Surgical removal of the inflamed tissue (see Figure 10.1) is called a tenosynovectomy. In RA, this type of surgery is most common in the wrist. This procedure is usually performed arthroscopically.

Osteotomy

An osteotomy (removal of bone) is rarely performed in RA; however, it may be an option if deformity of the bones adjacent to the joint becomes a problem.

Arthrodesis

Arthrodesis is the surgical fusing together of the two bones that meet to form a joint. The goal of the surgery is to eliminate joint movement, and as a result, eliminate pain, restore alignment, and increase joint stability. This type of surgery is most commonly done at the cervical and lumbar spine (the upper and lower parts of the spine), ankle, wrist, and fingers. The drawbacks of arthrodesis are the loss of movement and the resulting damage done to other joints that compensate for the loss of movement in the fused joint.

Arthroplasty

The term arthroplasty describes a more invasive surgical procedure, in which the orthopedic surgeon rebuilds or replaces joints that cannot be corrected by other types of surgery.

The first total joint replacements (TJR) were performed in the late 1950s by John Charnley.[5] With improvements in surgical techniques and materials over the last four decades of the twentieth century, the success rates for hip and knee replacements have risen to 90 percent or better.[6,7]

Based on a study published in 1998 that followed 1,600 people with RA over a twenty-three-year period,[8] one in four underwent TJR surgery, and one in eight had two joints replaced. Those with the most severe RA overall were the ones who needed a hip or knee replacement. When following up ten years later on those who had a joint replaced, 6 percent of knee replacements and 4 percent of hip replacements had to be redone.

Mechanical joints (prosthesis) are made up of two parts: one metal (stainless steel or alloys) and the other sturdy plastic. Prosthetics are secured into place one of two ways—either by fitting and locking the joint and bone together, or by using a plastic cement-like material to anchor the prosthesis into the bone. The location of the surgery, the artificial joint recipient's lifestyle, and the surgeon's preference, determine which method should be used.

The life span of an artificial joint replacement is highly individual, but they usually last anywhere from ten to twenty years. Factors that determine joint replacement longevity include a person's age, pre- and postoperative health, the amount of damage to the bone before surgery, lifestyle, type of joint used, and the surgical technique, among others. On average, people with RA have joint replacement surgery when they are ten years younger than people with osteoarthritis. As a result, they have the potential to live longer with an artificial joint,[9,10] which then increases their chances for complications to arise.

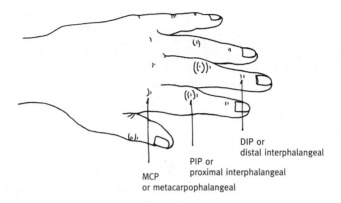

Fig. 10.2. Common sites for surgery in the hands.

COMMON AREAS FOR SURGERY

Hands and Wrists

There is little we do in a day that doesn't involve our hands and wrists, so it goes without saying that to lose function in these two areas is highly disruptive to a person's life. Rare is the person with RA—even mild RA—whose hands and wrists are not affected in some way by the disease.

As mentioned earlier in this chapter, the primary goals of any surgery are to reduce pain, correct deformities, and improve function. The most common sites for surgery in the hands (see Figure 10.2) are:

- the metacarpophalangeal (MCP) joints
- the proximal interphalangeal (PIP) joints
- the distal interphalangeal (DIP) joints

Synovectomies and tenosynovectomies are generally safe and effective surgical treatments when medication therapy or cortisone injections are ineffective at controlling inflammation. As well, reconstructing MCP joints is safe and reasonably effective at reducing pain and restoring some function to the hand. All three approaches can be done on an outpatient (no overnight stay required) basis.

In the wrist, joint replacements do not yet deliver consistent enough results. Surgical removal of damaged bone (osteotomy) or occasionally, fusing the bones together (arthrodesis) can provide good pain relief.

Shoulders and Elbows

RA doesn't affect the shoulder and elbow as often as it does other larger joints in the body (such as the knees and hips), but when it does, the pain can be just as unbearable and limit function as it does elsewhere.

The most common surgeries of the shoulder and elbow are arthroplasty, arthroscopic synovectomy, and tenosynovectomy. Because arthrodesis takes away a substantial percentage of the shoulder's ability to move, this procedure is only considered in individuals who have significant nerve damage of the deltoid and rotator cuff muscles, and those who have infection of the shoulder with loss of cartilage.

Because shoulder pain can travel to the elbow, surgery that effectively reduces pain and improves function in the shoulder may also take away pain and improve function in the elbow. Furthermore, as hand function is limited by elbow pain and stiffness, improved function in the elbow typically reduces pain and improves function in the hand.

Hips

For many with RA, surgery for hip pain and deformity can mean the difference between walking and not. For those over the age of fifty-five or sixty, total hip arthroplasty is the most common surgery today. It is successful approximately 90 percent of the time, and can last for up to ten to twenty years. Loosening remains the leading cause of long-term failure of hip replacements, but improvements in fixation of the artificial joint parts to bone has substantially improved over the years. Pain is the key symptom of hip replacement wear or loosening.

Surgeons are more reluctant to perform total hip arthroplasty in younger people or individuals who are more physically active because of uncertainty over how long it will last. However, the bottom line is function. Surgeons perform total joint replacements in individuals in their twenties when this is what is needed to keep them leading a productive and satisfying quality of life.

As explained earlier in this chapter, rehabilitation is essential to successful postsurgery results. Getting the muscles that surround the joint back into shape after surgery will bring back one's ability to carry on daily activities pain free, and in time, the ability to resume light-impact recreational activities such as golfing, swimming, bicycling, and walking.

Knees

The knee is perhaps the most abused joint in the human body, and because it is a complex structure that bears the weight of the body with each step it takes, it is particularly vulnerable to injury and general wear and tear.

The most commonly performed surgeries on the knee are arthroscopic surgery including synovectomy, total joint arthroplasty, and resurfacing arthroplasty (the latest development in knee surgery). Synovectomy is reasonably effective surgery for dealing with uncontrolled swelling of the synovial tissue lining the joint. Because these procedures can be done with limited disruption to the joint itself, it is usually performed as day surgery and recovery is rapid.

The results of total knee replacement are as stellar as those reported for the hip: Over 90 percent of people are still experiencing good results ten years after having their knee replaced. With a technique known as *resurfacing arthroplasty*, the surgeon resurfaces the ends of the femur, tibia, and sometimes, the patella bones, with metal and plastic, rather than replacing the entire knee joint. The supporting ligaments and tendon that surround the knee joint are left intact to help maintain stability and allow mobility.[11]

Osteotomy for knee arthritis is usually reserved for noninflammatory conditions, and as a result, is infrequently performed in people with RA.

Ankles and Feet

Problems of the ankles and feet are common in RA, and just like in other joints, they often need to be surgically treated when medication therapy, orthotics, splints, and the like are unsuccessful at controlling pain and the damage caused by the disease process.

Arthroscopy (to remove loose debris in the joints), osteotomy, and arthrodesis are the most common surgeries of the ankles and feet, but none offers permanent correction. The restriction of arthrodesis surgery for ankles and feet seems to deliver more desirable results for people than when performed in some of the other joints mentioned above. Surgery on toes can lead to dramatic pain relief.

Ankle joint arthritis can be managed with arthrodesis (fusion) or joint replacement. Despite some early failures with joint replacement of the ankle, evolution of designs and surgical technique continue to make this a viable option for the arthritic ankle.

GET EXPERT ADVICE

As with all the other parts of your treatment plan, getting expert advice from a surgeon and rheumatologist skilled in arthritis surgery and RA offer you the best chance for successful surgical results. While excellent guidelines and protocols exist, they will individualize a surgical treatment plan that caters to your specific needs.

Chapter 11

Pregnancy, Childbirth, and Menopause

"For each of us as women, there is a deep place within, where hidden and growing
our true spirit rises ... Within these deep places, each one holds
an incredible reserve of creativity and power ..."

—Audre Lorde

Conceiving a baby, growing it in the womb, giving birth, and raising a child can be some of the most fulfilling experiences life has to offer a woman—whether she has RA or not.

There's no doubt that you'll face challenges as a woman with RA, but moms who live with the disease and experts agree: If you want to have children, the rewards far outweigh the difficulties you may face. Your chances of becoming pregnant are normal, pregnancy will not make your disease worse, and your arthritis will not harm your baby, although there is a small possibility that RA will be passed along to your child through your genes and affect him or her later in life.

Before and during pregnancy, you and your rheumatologist may face tough decisions about medications, and 90 percent of women experience a flare in the three months after the baby is born (more on these topics later). But, all in all, pregnancy and childbirth are safe for both moms with RA, and their precious cargo.

Your Ability to Conceive

If you wish to have a baby, here's some good news: RA will not reduce your ability to conceive (your "fertility"). The disease can slightly increase the length of time it takes for the egg-meets-sperm miracle to occur (known as "fecundity"), but for most women who want to become pregnant, this doesn't pose an obstacle. Would-be moms may use this information to influence their decision to attempt to conceive sooner rather than later.

If you've heard that women with RA have a harder time getting pregnant, it's probably because studies done in 1957 and 1965 concluded that women with RA had fewer children, and therefore that they had lower fertility. What these studies ignored was that women may have chosen not to have children, especially in light of the fact that back then, doctors discouraged their female RA patients from having kids because the disease can be very severe, and effective treatments were not available at that time. Today, women with RA have about the same average number of children as women in the general population.

THE THREE RS OF PREGNANCY: RESPITE, RELIEF, AND REMISSION

One of the nicer side effects of carrying a baby is that you can get relief from the symptoms of RA. Doctors first made this link back in 1938, and since then, numerous studies have confirmed that 71 to 86 percent of women with RA experience disease improvement during pregnancy.[1,2,3] Only a small amount of research has been done on the degree of remission experienced, but results show that 50 to 65 percent of women with RA go into complete remission during pregnancy. However, 20 to 30 percent of pregnant women with RA continue to have active disease.

Nature has some wonderful ways. Women whose symptoms do improve tend to experience relief during the first trimester (first three months) of their pregnancy,[4] when nausea, vomiting, and fatigue are usually at their worst. That relief is often sustained, or gets even better, as the pregnancy progresses. There's plenty of individual variation, though—some women don't experience relief until their last three months of pregnancy. Women whose RA improves during one pregnancy usually get improvement in other pregnancies as well.[5,6]

Unfortunately, it is almost impossible to predict whether you'll be one of the women for whom pregnancy provides a respite from RA. The course your disease will take while you're growing a baby cannot be predicted by your age, the severity of your RA, your degree of disability, the length of time you've had RA,[7] the sex of your baby, or the presence of a positive rheumatoid factor blood test (see Chapter 2 for a discussion of rheumatoid factor). What we do know is that for the vast majority of women, RA symptoms do not get any worse during pregnancy.

BEST ODDS FOR A HEALTHY, HAPPY PREGNANCY

Before Becoming Pregnant

The most important medical things to consider before becoming pregnant are the length of time prior to conception that certain medications should be stopped, and the need for supplemental vitamins.

For example, a relationship has been established between insufficient amounts of maternal folic acid and an increased risk for babies born with spina bifida. Therefore, it is recommended that all women (not just those with RA) considering pregnancy take 400 mcg of folic acid daily for at least three months prior to conception, and continue to take this supplement during pregnancy.

See your rheumatologist as soon as you know that you want to start trying to conceive—ideally, six months before you want to conceive—so that the two of you can devise an appropriate and safe medication therapy plan. (Men who wish to impregnate their partners should do the same, by the way.) Less than half of all pregnancies are planned, however, so if you have an accidental pregnancy, don't worry—but do see your rheumatologist as soon as you know. You might also wish to review the "Medications During Pregnancy" section of this chapter.

Some rheumatologists recommend that women wait until they are in relative remission before getting pregnant, so they'll cope better with the physical demands of pregnancy and medications can more easily be reduced.

Choose a Great Caregiver

When possible, it's best to consult with a pregnancy caregiver (registered/certified midwife, physician) prior to attempting to conceive, so that you can develop a plan specific to your own body that will support a healthy pregnancy. Your rheumatologist will also play an important role in planning your medication therapy before, during, and after the pregnancy (more on this later).

Give serious thought to who would you like to have support you through your pregnancy and your baby's birth. Where would you like your baby to be born? Who would you like to have present? What kind of atmosphere would you prefer? Take the time to make decisions on these and other specific choices you'll need to make during labor and birthing.

Pre-Natal Nutrition

Eating well is essential to a healthy pregnancy and baby. Inadequate amounts and quality of nutrition are strongly related to low birthweight babies, who are at significant risk for birth defects, illness, and developmental problems. If possible, visit a registered dietitian to get a nutritional assessment based on your current diet, and from there, a nutritional plan unique to you. In general, if a woman is not medically underweight or undernourished prior to conception, her usual food intake levels are considered adequate for the first twenty weeks of pregnancy. After that, she needs to begin to increase her protein and caloric intake based on her weight and frame.

Exercise

The amount and type of physical activity you do can have a significant helpful effect for the mother and her baby, both short term and long term. Exercise can help relieve backache, prevent urinary incontinence, condition your body for labor, and stimulate baby—positively affecting her growth. Each woman should get specific exercise advice from an RA-wise physical therapist (if she has one) or her rheumatologist. However, in general, do not strain during exercise, do not get overheated (hot tubs and saunas are a definite no-no), and at minimum, maintain the level of exercise you were doing prior to pregnancy. If you were not exercising prior to becoming pregnant, start out easily and gradually develop a more strenuous exercise program. See Chapter 5 for a guide to exercising with RA.

Lovemaking

It's okay for a woman to make love, including sexual intercourse, during pregnancy if she so desires—unless she is experiencing specific medical problems. During the third trimester, for example, women with premature ripening of the cervix or a history of third trimester problems may be advised against having intercourse: talk with your caregiver.

Preparing for Childbirth

Decide which approach to childbirth most appeals to you, and then take childbirth classes. Advance information makes women feel more comfortable during their labor and better able to cope with the experience. Also, review our section on Caesarian births later in this chapter, just in case.

Useful books on pregnancy include: *Birthing From Within: An Extra-Ordinary Guide to Childbirth Preparation* by Pam England and Rob Horowitz; *The Pregnant Woman's Comfort Book: A Self-Nurturing Guide to Your Emotional Well-Being During Pregnancy and Early Motherhood* by Jennifer Louden; and Sheila Kitzinger's *Your Baby, Your Way: Making Pregnancy Decisions and Birth Plans*.

WILL RA CAUSE PREGNANCY COMPLICATIONS?

According to the multitude of reliable studies done over the past thirty years, women with RA are *not* at a higher risk of having pregnancy complications such as gestational hypertension (a pregnancy-induced condition in which the mother gets high blood pressure, leading to reduced blood flow and problems for the baby, and, rarely, severe problems for the mother such as liver failure and cerebral hemorrhages); spontaneous abortion (miscarriage); intrauterine growth restriction (a condition in which the baby is undersized—either all over its body or everywhere except the head and heart); premature labor (starting labor before twenty-eight weeks of gestation), or low birthweight babies (under 5.5 pounds or 2,500 grams).[8] Women with RA are also not at a higher risk for requiring Caesarian births.

However, it may be worth noting that a recent study in Norway came to conclusions that contradict the above generally agreed on information from the past three decades. The study, conducted in 1998, examined all of births in Norway between 1967 and 1995. It found increased rates of preeclampsia, premature birth, Caesarian births, and low birthweight babies in a combined category of women with RA and women with ankylosing spondylitis. This single study needs to be repeated, however, before medical opinion will be swayed.

DISEASE ACTIVITY AFTER THE BABY IS BORN

Almost all women with RA—approximately ninety percent—experience a disease recurrence within three to four months of giving birth or otherwise ending a pregnancy. The timing of such flares is not related to when a woman begins to menstruate again. Please don't wait for a flare before seeing your rheumatologist after childbirth. About four to six weeks after the baby is born, visit your rheumatologist so they can examine you for signs of an imminent flare and make recommendations.

One 1996 study did find a relationship between more severe RA and women who conceived many children, breast-fed larger numbers of children, and breast-fed for longer periods of time. However, most of the small amount of research available suggests that having a baby does not affect how your disease will progress over the long term, regardless of your number of pregnancies or whether these pregnancies end through childbirth, spontaneous abortion, or termination.

Breast-feeding

For women with RA, breast-feeding can create ambivalent feelings. On the one hand, breast-feeding can be hard on the shoulders and arms, and a singular research study has suggested a possible relationship between breast-feeding and more severe RA. On the other hand, no person-made formula can approximate the perfect food produced in a mother's milk. The benefits of breast-feeding to the baby are incontrovertible, and include such things as baby's increased immunity, decreased risk of gastrointestinal infections, ear infections, allergies, and certain cancers, and mom's quicker return to prepregnancy weight and tone.

If you feel determined to breast-feed but joint pain or limited range of motion make it too difficult for you to hold baby as you need to for breast-feeding, you might consider seeing an occupational therapist and/or lactation consultant for suggestions.

In reality, though, it may be difficult for some women with RA to continue to breast-feed once a postpartum flare strikes. The need for medication therapy, coupled with pain and joint problems, gets in the way of their ability to breast-feed, and they find that it's a relief when they stop. Please don't punish yourself if this is the case for you. Remember that more than anything, your baby needs a happy, healthy mama—and you need and deserve to have a positive early experience of being her mother. Consult your care provider for advice on the best formula for baby. Many excellent ones are available today and have been effective in meeting the nutritional needs of countless thriving bundles of joy.

In preparation for the possibility that you'll need to stop breast-feeding early, you might wish to pump and store a good supply of breastmilk for later, as well as accustom baby to taking a bottle. The ideal time to introduce the bottle is between baby's third and fifth weeks of life. Research shows that introducing the bottle earlier may cause "nipple confusion," and baby may begin to refuse the breast. If you wait until after baby's fifth week, she may refuse to take the bottle at all.

CAESARIAN BIRTH

All women and their babies are at some risk for needing a Caesarian birth; however, there is no evidence that women with RA need Caesarian births more often than other women.

Having no choice but to give birth through Caesarian can be disappointing for women who have an emotional or spiritual investment in experiencing vaginal childbirth. Others welcome a planned Caesarian birth without going through labor at all. With preparation and planning, many women have had beautiful Caesarian birth experiences. Books such as *The Well Pregnancy Book* can help you prepare physically and emotionally for giving birth to your child the high-tech way, and for the six-week recovery period that follows.

A word of caution about Caesarian births for women with RA: if your disease involves your cervical spine or your cricoarytenoid joint, general anesthesia could carry an increased risk.[9] This is because advanced disease can lead to loosening in your cervical spine, so that when your neck is moved backward to place a breathing tube in your throat, your spinal cord is compressed. This would be rare, but also extremely dangerous if it occurred (it can cause death). If you have a Caesarian birth, be sure to inform the surgeon and the anesthetist that you have RA, and inform them that caution is needed with your neck.

Fortunately, the need for general anesthesia in childbirth is rare. It occurs in unplanned Caesarian births, when the baby is in significant distress and there isn't enough time for the delicate process of administering an epidural anesthetic into the spine. Most women with RA who have Caesarian births can receive an epidural anesthetic, which enables them to stay awake during the birth of their baby.

MEDICATIONS DURING PREGNANCY

"How will medications affect my baby?" is a major—and understandable—concern for virtually all pregnant women.

Let's look at the positive side, first: you could be among the large group of women (three-quarters) who require no RA drugs during at least some part of their pregnancy, thanks to a pregnancy-induced reduction in your symptoms, or even a complete remission. However, some rheumatologists do recommend that women with RA stay on medication even during the absence of symptoms, to reduce the risk and severity of a flare after the baby is born.[10] Of course, 20 to 30 percent of women with RA do not experience relief from symptoms during pregnancy, and usually need to continue taking medications throughout the pregnancy.

For these women, there is mixed news. Scientists don't yet have all the answers about how RA medications affect the growing fetus. What they do know is that almost every drug crosses the placenta. Occasionally placental enzymes cause medications to change (sometimes into less toxic substances) once they're inside the placenta.[11] Nonetheless, many women with RA have become pregnant and have required medications for their RA, and there have been no problems whatsoever.

In the past, patients and physicians have relied on the categorization of drugs according to U.S. Food and Drug Administration criteria.[12] However, these are undergoing changes and the A, B, C, and D classification will almost certainly disappear. Much of the information on drugs in pregnancy is complex and is being updated all the time. On the following pages, you'll find information about the safety of specific RA drugs during pregnancy and breast-feeding. The information is provided to help you to ask the right questions. If you have questions about any of these drugs, we strongly recommend that you discuss them with your rheumatologist, or with one of the recognized international centers that specialize in drugs and pregnancy—yes, there are people who devote their entire lives to the study of drug safety during pregnancy and breast feeding (see Chapter 12). As with every other aspect of your health care, make sure you are talking to an expert who has up-to-date information.

The terminology of pregnancy includes the following: "First trimester" refers to the first three months after conception; "second trimester" or "mid-trimester" refers to months 4, 5, and 6; and "third trimester" or "final trimester" refers to months 7, 8, and 9. Most of the body organs develop during the first third of pregnancy (e.g., heart, lungs, liver, kidneys, and so on). The big exception is the brain, which develops throughout pregnancy. Thus, if a drug has an increased risk of causing cleft lip in the fetus, this would only be a risk if the medication was consumed in the first three months of the pregnancy. If the drug was needed to treat the RA, it could be taken after month 3 without any increase in the risk of cleft lip. In contrast, a medication that can affect the brain and crosses the barrier between the brain and the rest of the body would be of concern throughout pregnancy.

While not as much is known about the safety of medications during pregnancy as one would like, it is important to know that many of the ones used by nonpregnant RA patients have been used without problem during pregnancy. In fact, for a woman to spend months in severe pain, day and night, unable to move about or stay fit, is likely not at all good for a fetus. The psyche affects every other aspect of human development and health, and it is likely to affect the fetus. A happy active pregnant woman should be the goal, and it may require multiple medications in many women with RA, at least for a portion of the pregnancy.

Information on arthritis medications and breast-feeding is more limited than for pregnancy. It is known that for most drugs, only 2 percent of the drug per pound of the mother ends up in the baby. Thus, if a one hundred-pound woman takes one thousand units of a medication (ten units per pound), the ten-pound baby will ingest 2/100ths of that or 0.2 units per pound during breast-feeding. This is certainly reassuring. However, many women may not be able to breast-feed or may have to stop breast-feeding early because of the medications they need to control their RA. While breast-feeding confers early immunity and other benefits on the newborn baby, it must be remembered that many of the reports of problems with breast-feeding come from developing countries, where things as simple as being able to provide noninfected water may play an overwhelming role in infant health or lack of it. Current formulas for bottle feeding are excellent and should be a real option for a mother with RA who requires medications that preclude breastfeeding. Given the very high frequency of flare ups in RA after having a baby, this will be an important topic for many mothers to consider and discuss with their health team members.

Specific Medications

Comments on a selected group of medications that someone with RA might need while considering pregnancy or subsequent breast-feeding follows. It is not meant as a textbook on what is one of the most complicated and controversial areas of medication therapy but, rather, as a guide that may help you to ask the right questions. We encourage everyone contemplating pregnancy to discuss this with their rheumatologist and GP.

- **Misoprostol (Cytotec):** This medication acts to protect the stomach from side effects of nonsteroidal anti-inflammatory drugs. It can be used with any of these drugs and is sometimes available as a fixed combination (e.g., diclofenac plus misoprostol is sold as Arthrotec®). The drug may induce abortion and should be stopped when one starts trying to become pregnant. Very rarely, misoprostol can cause a malformation called moefius, which includes paralysis of the main nerve to the face. Of course, it is not used during pregnancy either.

- **Analgesics:** Among all of the medications used by people with RA, acetaminophen appears to be the safest for both pregnancy and breast-feeding. There has been considerable experience with this medication and, if pain is a problem, the use of acetaminophen is likely as close to being safe as is possible.

- **Nonsteroidal Anti-Inflammatory Drugs (NSAIDs):** As with all classes of drugs in which there are many different chemical compounds, the most information on safety exists for those that have been used the longest. There are more than a dozen NSAIDs and the number continues to increase. The oldest drug is aspirin. There have been dozens of studies on aspirin and no increase in malformations has been found. In that many pregnant women with RA do require NSAIDs, especially early on in the pregnancy, there is a tendency to rely on older drugs such as aspirin, ibuprofen and naproxen. However, all of the NSAIDs are likely similar. The evidence to date is that when one compares women with RA who take NSAIDs to those who do not take NSAIDs, the pregnancy outcomes, the duration of labor and the frequency of complications at childbirth are similar.[13] Also, the babies are just as healthy. No NSAID has been shown to cause birth defects.

   Because NSAIDs work by affecting prostaglandin synthesis, they can affect an important valve in the circulation called the *ductus arteriosus*, so that it closes too early. This closure is rare and always occurs in the final phase of a pregnancy. Because of this, it is reasonable for the individual with RA to try to stop or decrease the NSAID during the third trimester. Fortunately, RA often improves during pregnancy and the improvement is greatest in the final third of pregnancy. If NSAIDs must be continued, it may be worth seeking a consultation with a cardiologist specializing in fetal echocardiography, so that the ductus arteriosus can be monitored by ultrasound.

   Small amounts of NSAIDs do enter the breast milk. Short half-life NSAIDs such as ibuprofen and diclofenac may be preferred, but problems have not been reported with any of the NSAIDs when the baby is healthy.

- **Corticosteroids** (e.g., prednisone, methylprednisolone, dexamethasone, triamcinolone): Corticosteroids have generally been considered safe for the fetus and for breast-feeding a newborn baby. Traditionally, they have been the preferred powerful medication in women with active arthritis. Fortunately, usually only low doses (prednisone 10 mg/day or less) are needed. It has recently been reported that if corticosteroids are used, there may be a small risk of an increase in the frequency of cleft lip and cleft palate in the child. Use of corticosteroids appears to triple this risk.[14] However, it must be kept in mind that the background risk of cleft lip or cleft palate is only 1 in 1,000, so that tripling the risk increases it to only 3 in 1,000. Not only is the chance of this happening low, but cleft lip or cleft palate are now completely correctable surgically. Because the cleft is closed by the end of the first third of pregnancy—remember that most organs except the brain are developed by the end of the first third of the pregnancy—the use of corticosteroids after this period should cause no increase in risk whatsoever.

  There has also been a single report of a corticosteroid called *dexamethasone*, that is given to mothers whose baby may be born very early, possibly affecting the IQ of the child. Despite extensive use of corticosteroids during the pregnancies of women with RA, no such effect has been noted. Clearly more studies will be done on this in the coming years.

  Corticosteroids continue to be the safest of the powerful medications for use in pregnancy and are considered safe for breast-feeding. The American Academy of Pediatrics considers corticosteroids compatible with breastfeeding[15,16,17,18] in doses of less than 20 mg/day.

- **Hydroxychloroquine:** It has recently been learned that the half-life of the antimalarial, hydroxychloroquine, is forty days—the half-life is the time it takes for half the drug to be metabolized to an inactive substance. This means it will take about two hundred days to clear the medication from the body after it has been stopped. Thus, a great many women who became pregnant while taking hydroxychloroquine had a considerable amount of it present during much of their pregnancy. Also, a great many women have taken this class of drugs while pregnant to prevent malaria and no increase in congenital malformations has been seen. Although the dose used to prevent malaria is lower than to treat RA, the fact that no increase in congenital malformations has been reported is reassuring.

The decision to stop taking hydroxychloroquine prior to pregnancy is probably best discussed with a rheumatologist or an expert in medications and pregnancy. Many rheumatologists consider that it is safe to continue hydroxychlorquine during pregnancy where the RA requires treatment with a disease modifying medication.

Only about 2 percent of hydroxychloroquine is secreted in breast milk. While the drug can accumulate in the baby, follow-up of infants of mothers breast-feeding while taking hydroxychloroquine have shown no abnormalities in the eyes compared to babies whose mothers had not received the medication. As with pregnancy, this appears to be one of the safest disease modifying medications to use during breast-feeding.

Far and away, the greatest risk from hydroxychloroquine comes if an infant or toddler consumes hydroxychloroquine as a tablet. As little as a single pill may kill an infant. Thus, please make certain that the hydroxychloroquine bottle is never available to an infant or toddler. If you don't have children at home, think of grandchildren, neighbors' children, and others who may be at risk if they visit.

- **Sulfasalazine:** This is another medication that is frequently used in mild RA. In more severe disease, it is used in combination with methotrexate or methotrexate and hydroxychloroquine. In the past, the FDA has been concerned about the use of sulfasalazine, particularly in the third trimester. However, in persons with inflammatory bowel disease, another autoimmune condition in which the medication is effective, sulfasalazine has been found to be safe for both pregnancy and breast-feeding[19,20,21]. It is generally felt that sulfasalazine can be used in RA pregnancy where the clinical situation suggests a disease modifying medication is needed. With breast-feeding, rare side effects have occurred on the liver and blood system of babies missing the G6PD enzyme, as small amounts of sulfasalazine is passed in the breast milk. A baby can be tested for this presence of the G6PD enzyme.
- **Minocycline:** Tetracyclines are not given during pregnancy or breast-feeding, as they can affect the teeth of the fetus and baby. It is not certain that this occurs with the newer tetracyclines such as minocyline. However, this drug is often used for mild disease for which there are drugs such as hydroxychloroquine that may suffice.
- **Gold Salts** (auranofin, gold thiomalate, gold thioglucose): There have been some suggestions that newborn babies exposed to gold have an increased risk of liver or blood side effects. However,

there is no increased risk of congenital malformations when exposure occurs during the first trimester—the high risk period.[22,23,24] Some rheumatologists consider gold safe during pregnancy, although they are less likely to recommend breast-feeding.

- **D-Penicillamine:** D-penicillamine is generally not used during pregnancy. There have been reports of *cutis laxa* (babies with loose skin) in up to 5 percent of fetuses exposed to the drug.
- **Methotrexate:** Methotrexate has an antifolate effect (that is why folic acid is used to prevent side effects when methotrexate is used) and it is known that a deficiency of folic acid in the first third of pregnancy is associated with the development of a congenital anomaly, neural tube defects in the spinal cord. This is the reason that women are encouraged to take a folic acid vitamin supplement prior to actually becoming pregnant. While there is no evidence that methotrexate in the low doses used in rheumatoid arthritis actually cause malformations, it is known that high doses are a potent cause of abortion and congenital malformations.[25] Thus, for both women planning to conceive and men who wish to impregnate their partner, the current practice is to suggest that methotrexate be stopped three months or more ahead of the conception.[26]

  It is not clear that methotrexate is fully immunosuppressive. But, because immunosuppressive drugs may increase the risk of cancer in the child, there is reluctance to recommend breast-feeding if methotrexate is used.[27]
- **Leflunomide:** This new agent causes congenital malformations in animals at a blood level that is much lower than the blood level achieved in humans. Thus, it is not given to women for whom there is any chance of becoming pregnant. Also, the drug is metabolized very slowly so that if pregnancy is considered, the drug must be removed from the woman or the man using a special treatment protocol with cholestyramine or activated charcoal. Once this has been done, the absence of the drug from the blood must be confirmed by a test for the drug in a blood sample.
- **Immunosuppressive Drugs:** The major immunosuppressive medications that are used to treat severe RA include azathioprine, cyclosporin-A, and cyclophosphamide. There is a theoretical concern that if a fetus or infant is exposed to these drugs, there may be an increase in the risk of developing cancer as an adult. Understandably, this is very difficult to study. One would have to assemble a large group of individuals who had been exposed to the immunosuppressive drug during pregnancy or breast-feeding,

then follow them for ten, twenty, or even more years. Based on what we do know, it is believed that the risk would be small for azathioprine and cyclosporin-A and higher for cyclophosphamide. Unfortunately, use of an immunosuppressive medication may not be optional for some women with RA who become pregnant. Many rheumatologists would not encourage breastfeeding when an immunosuppressive medication is used, as this clearly is optional.

- **Azathioprine:** Among the immunosuppressive medications, there is the most information about this one. The drug may be partially metabolized by the placenta, thereby reducing the amount that reaches the fetus. There have been no reports of increased risk of congenital malformations and fertility has not been compromised. There is considerable experience with this drug in pregnant women who have had an organ transplant (e.g., kidney transplant), and there is no evidence that it is dangerous, based on the information actually available. Women taking azathioprine require monthly monitoring during the final trimester to check the levels of their blood cells including the platelets (if the blood cell count is low, the dose of azathioprine is reduced). Some babies have been born with low white blood cell counts and low platelet counts because of the medication (this makes the babies potentially vulnerable to infection and bleeding problems).[28] Breastfeeding would not be encouraged because of the immunosuppressive nature of the medication.

- **Cyclosporin-A:** This medication crosses the placenta and enters the baby's circulation, although in the newborn baby, the level decreases to zero within a couple of days.[29,30] Like azathioprine, this drug has been used widely in organ transplantation. No effect on fertility and no increase risk of congenital malformations has been detected. Breast-feeding would not be encouraged because of the immunosuppressive nature of the medication and the at least theoretical risk of cancer in the child.[31]

- **Cyclophosphamide:** This medication can permanently reduce the ability of both men and women to have children (fertility is reduced) and it can cause congenital malformation.[32] It is sometimes necessary to use the medication during pregnancy when the health of the mother is at risk. Some normal healthy babies have been born whose mothers had received this medication during pregnancy. Use of this agent would require careful discussion with individuals expert in the use of medications in pregnancy. Cyclophosphamide should be discontinued several months prior to a planned conception. Breast-feeding would not be advised.[33] Chlo-

rambucil, a drug similar to cyclophosphamide, is rarely used but
has similar side effects and risks.[34]
- **Anti-TNF Alpha Drugs:** There is no information available as yet
  on etanercept or inflixamab. Major international research centers
  focusing on medications in pregnancy will no doubt be collecting
  information (see Chapter 12).

Caring For Baby

During a pregnancy-induced remission, most women with RA feel better
than they have in years, and many forget how painful and debilitating RA
can really be. It's wise to prepare yourself both emotionally and from a
practical standpoint for when the inevitable postpartum flare occurs. Here
are some tips:

- Stock your freezer with nutritious, microwavable meals *before* the
  baby comes.
- Find the most RA-friendly way to diaper baby. Some women
  whose RA affects their hands find the sticky tabs on disposable
  diapers too difficult to manage. Washable diapers pose laundry-
  related challenges, unless you can afford a diaper service. If you
  do go that route, avoid diapers that employ snaps or pins—Velcro
  fasteners are probably easiest on your hands.
- Prepare yourself psychologically for the possibility that you may
  need assistance taking care of baby from time to time; that you
  may be unable to breast-feed baby due to shoulder pain or medication therapy; that your house may not be as tidy or clean as
  you'd like for a while; and that caring for yourself and baby may
  be all that you can do for a period of months.
- Plan to have help with the baby. Do you have a friend or relative
  who could come to stay with you for a few weeks, perhaps on
  short notice, if or when the flare strikes? Or a couple of friends
  who might each commit to helping out for a few hours each week?
  Most people love to help with baby, and just need to be asked.
- Prepare others in your life to expect less of you when the baby
  comes. Even for women who don't have RA, caring for a newborn
  or infant is overwhelming. You'll need to focus on yourself and
  the baby for a while, and let the rest of the world go by (unless
  they want to help, of course).
- Stock up on baby clothes that are easy to put on and fasten—and
  ask the same of others who wish to give baby gifts. Snaps are out;
  zippers and Velcro are in. Buy shoes with Velcro fasteners rather
  than laces.

- Set up baby's change table so that everything is within easy reach.
- Consider having someone make you a trolley, so that you can push baby from place to place, rather than carrying baby with painful shoulders, hands, and arms. Some strollers can work well for this purpose as well—keep that in mind when you go shopping for yours.
- Call your occupational therapist when you bring baby home. Your OT may be able to make a home visit and give you a wealth of energy-saving, joint-protecting suggestions.

For more general tips and information on optimizing your environment and energy use, see Chapter 9.

MENOPAUSE

Research has not shown a difference between the effects of menopause between women with RA and those in the general population. However, women with RA are more likely to develop osteoporosis.

This is likely due to decreased amounts of exercise, and use of corticosteroids. Factors that influence the degree of osteoporosis include disease activity, immobility, age, and menopause.

The effect that corticosteroids (such as prednisone) have on osteoporosis is controversial, with some researchers finding that cumulative use increases osteoporosis, and others finding no effect on osteoporosis.[35,36,37] All in all, however, corticosteroids probably do cause bone loss.[38,39] (See Chapter 6 for a discussion of osteoporosis).

Hormone replacement therapy, or HRT, can be used to treat many symptoms associated with menopause (as well as osteoporosis), although its use is controversial because of side effects and differing opinions and data about how well it works.[40] However, if you have osteoporosis, the benefits of estrogen therapy probably outweigh the risks.

Some studies specifically investigating the use of HRT on bone mineral density of postmenopausal women with RA found that HRT prevented further bone loss or actually improved bone density. HRT was recommended as a valuable addition to conventional antirheumatic therapy.

THE PILL

Although researchers are divided on the subject, many are convinced that to at least some extent, use of oral contraceptives ("the pill") by healthy women makes the development of RA less likely, or among women destined to develop RA, postpones the onset of the disease or makes it less severe.[41,42]

In one study, women who have not used oral contraceptives *and* have not had any children are four times more likely to develop RA than women who have either had a child or used oral contraceptives.[43]

PREGNANCY, BREAST-FEEDING, AND ONSET OF RA

Pregnancy and RA Onset

It is unlikely that a woman will develop RA for the first time during pregnancy (the risk is about one in 16,000),[44,45,46,47] but there is a definite increase in the risk of developing RA in the postpartum period (up to five times more likely than in other periods of her life). This is especially true in the first three months after giving birth, and especially with the first baby.[48] Since something clearly suppresses RA during pregnancy, it is perhaps not surprising that RA onset also is often supressed until after a baby is born. A baby's sex does not affect whether its mother will develop RA after pregnancy.[49]

There are many reasons to suspect that hormones found predominantly in females (such as estrogen) are responsible for RA: an increased frequency of RA in females, symptom relief during pregnancy, symptom changes during the menstrual cycle, and symptom reoccurrence following pregnancy. Unfortunately, although the role of hormones such as estrogen continue to be investigated, they clearly do not explain the entire RA puzzle.

With regard to the improvement of RA during pregnancy, one promising hypothesis has to do with the markers on each of our cells called human leukocyte antigens (HLA). The baby's cells are composed of DNA from both its mother and father. While the baby is growing in the uterus, it sloughs some of its cells, which then enter its mother's blood stream. Thus, some of the genetic information from the father mixes in the blood of the baby's mother. Research is suggesting that when the HLAs sloughed by the baby contain genetic information that is incompatible with the mother's genetic information, there is a more favorable RA outcome.[50,51,52] That is, when the difference between mother and fetus was greatest, remission of the woman's RA was more likely. Further research is being carried out to see if these results can be repeated.

Breast-feeding and RA Onset

Some researchers have suggested that onset of RA is related to breast-feeding.[53,54,55,56,57,58,59] They believe that the hormone prolactin, which is at high levels when women are nursing, makes the body more susceptible to inflammation. Animal studies have shown that when the gland that secretes prolactin is removed, research animals do not develop arthritis. In addition, a substance called bromocriptine, which blocks prolactin, also appears to block the development of arthritis in animals. Further study is needed.

Chapter 12

MORE RESOURCES

"If you don't know where you are going, you'll probably end up someplace else."

—*Yogi Berra*

Your PLAN TO WIN involves learning everything you can about RA. By reading this book, you've taken a giant leap forward in your understanding of the disease process, and you've gained a vast amount of knowledge about how you, personally, can influence your symptoms and prevent joint damage.

A book such as this one aims to provide information and tools in many areas: from lifestyle to medications, exercise, relationships, sex, mind-body work, nutrition, reproductive health, and surgery. As such, it can only scratch the surface of many of these topics. We have drawn on hundreds of studies, reports, books, and experts worldwide to provide you with the most reliable, up-to-date information, but there is always more to be learned.

If you wish to expand your knowledge of a specific topic, seek emotional support, involve yourself in advocacy efforts, or get a referral to an RA health professional, the following credible, tried, and true resources may be of assistance.

A special note on websites: We have provided a list of arthritis and RA-specific sites that we feel provide reliable information and are linked with credible organizations. New sites pop up daily, of course, so you'll need to exercise caution when you venture onto the internet on your own. Ask yourself: Does this site promote a particular product or therapy? If the site makes medical claims, are these claims scientifically researched and referenced? Does a credible organization or rheumatic disease specialist back this site?

Also, be aware that website addresses (known as URLs) change constantly. If you type in an address and receive an error message, don't assume the site is no longer functional. It may be down temporarily, or it may have moved, so try entering key words from the site's title—for example, "Arthritis Foundation"—in the search feature of an Internet search engine.

ASSOCIATIONS FOR PEOPLE WITH ARTHRITIS

The following not-for-profit groups exist to represent and serve the needs of people with any of the one hundred or more forms of arthritis. Each is different in terms of its activities and services, but in general they may offer some or all of the following: free brochures on arthritis and its management; names of local rheumatologists and health professionals who specialize in treating people with various forms of arthritis—including RA; toll-free telephone information and support; support groups; exercise classes; advocacy; and opportunities to get involved in raising awareness and funds for arthritis research and care. Contact the national office to find out how to get in touch with the chapter nearest you.

Australia

The Arthritis Foundation of Australia
GPO Box 121
Sydney, NSW 2000
Telephone: +61 2 9552 6085
Website: www.info@arthritisfoundation.com.au

Canada

The Arthritis Society
393 University Avenue, Suite 1700
Toronto, Ontario M5G 1E6
Telephone: (416) 979-7228
Toll free: 1-800-321-1433
Email: info@arthritis.ca
Website: www.arthritis.ca

New Zealand

Arthritis Foundation of New Zealand (Inc.)
Ninth Floor, 169 The Terrace, Box 10-202
Wellington
New Zealand
Telephone: 04-472-1427
Fax: 04-472-7066
Website: www.arthritis.org.nz

United Kingdom

Arthritis Care has chapters in England, Northern Ireland, Scotland, and Wales. For information, contact:

Arthritis Care
18 Stephenson Way
London, NW1 2HD
United Kingdom
Telephone: 020 7380 6500
Helpline: 080 8800 4050 (free) 12.00-16.00 week days
Publications: 0845 600 6868
020 7380 6555 (standard rates) 10.00-16.00 week days
Fax: 020 7380 6505
Website: www.arthritis.bocc.net

United States of America

The Arthritis Foundation
P.O. Box 7669
Atlanta, GA
30357-0669
USA
Telephone: (404) 872-7100
Toll free: 1-800-283-7800
Email: help@arthritis.org
Website: www.arthritis.org

International: Arthritis and Rheumatism International (ARI)

This is an association of national organizations whose members are, principally, people whose lives are affected by arthritis. Its mission is to provide a forum for the worldwide exchange of knowledge and experiences among organizations of people affected by arthritis, and to strengthen their voice through worldwide cooperation. Its objective is to improve the quality of life of people with arthritis.

In the United States, call: (404) 965-7540. For more information, visit the American Arthritis Foundation website or contact the current president of ARI:

Per-aage Bjoerke
Norsk Reumatikerforbund
Prof. Dahls
gt. 32, Box 2653
N-0203 Oslo, Norway
Telephone: (47) 22-54-7600

ARTHRITIS—GENERAL

Books

Arthritis: Your Complete Exercise Guide, Neil F. Gordon, The Cooper Clinic & Research Institute. IL: Human Kinetics Publ., 1993. ISBN 0-87322-392-6

Be Sick Well: A Healthy Approach to Chronic Illness, by Jeff Kane. CA: New Harbinger Publications, 1991. ISBN 1-879-23708-3

Mayo Clinic on Chronic Pain, by David W. Swanson, M.D. (Editor-in-Chief). New York: Kensington, 1999. ISBN 1-893005-02-X

No More Sleepless Nights, by Peter Hauri and Shirley Linde. Toronto: John Wiley & Sons, 1996 (revised ed.). ISBN 0-471-14904-7

Pain: Learning to Live Without It, by David Corey. Toronto: Macmillan Canada, 1993 (revised ed.). ISBN 0-771-59199-3

The Arthritis Helpbook: A Tested Self-Management Program for Coping with Arthritis and Fibromyalgia, by Kate Lorig and James Fries. Cambridge, MA: Perseus, 2000. ISBN 0-7382-0224-X

The Arthritis Foundation's Guide to Alternative Therapies, by Judith Horstman. Marietta, GA: Longstreet Press, 1999. ISBN 0-912423-23-4

The Essential Arthritis Cookbook, by Sarah L. Morgan. MN: Appletree Press, 1995. ISBN 0-9620471-6-3

Walk with Ease: Your Guide for Walking for Better Health, Improved Fitness and Less Pain, Atlanta, GA: The Arthritis Foundation, 1999. ISBN 0-912423-22-6

Magazines

Arthritis News
Published quarterly by The Arthritis Society (Canada) and Rogers Media. Features intelligent, well-written articles to help understand and deal with arthritis, including information on latest research and treatment, strategies for outsmarting the disease, and interviews with experts.

Arthritis News/Rogers Media
777 Bay Street, 5th Floor
Toronto, Ontario
M5W 1A7
Toll free: 1-800-217-0591
Or read/search *Arthritis News* online at www.arthritis.ca

Arthritis Today
Published by The Arthritis Foundation (United States) six times per year. Offers reliable information on a variety of topics, including the latest news about arthritis research, medications, alternative therapies, exercise, self-help tips, and more.

British Society for Rheumatology
41 Eagle Street
London WC1R 4AR
United Kingdom
Tel. 020 7242 3313
Fax. 020 7242 3277
E-mail: bsr@rheumatology.org.uk
Website: www.rheumatology.org.uk

Canadian Rheumatology Association (CRA)
The CRA mailing address and phone number changes every two years with
the appointment of the association's president, thus you will need to con-
tact this group through their website or email address, or you can contact
The Arthritis Society's office (see listing on page 222) for the information.
E-mail: crawebmaster@maci.mccaig.ucalgary.ca
Website: www.cra.ucalgary.ca

Arthritis Health Professionals' Associations

These national associations represent nonphysician health professionals
who specialize in rheumatology, such as: nurses, physiotherapists, occupational therapists, sociologists, psychologists, podiatrists, and educators.

AUSTRALIA

Rheumatology Health Professionals Association
Goatcher Clinical Research Unit
SCGH
C Block 1st Floor
Hospital Ave
Nedlands 6009 WA
Telephone: 08 9346 2158
E-mail: enquiresausrhpa.com
Website: www.ausrhpa.com

UNITED KINGDOM

British Health Professionals in Rheumatology
c.o. British Society for Rheumatology
41 Eagle Street
London
WC 1 R 4A
Telephone:+44 (0) 20 7242 3313,
Fax:+44 (0) 20 7242 3277
E-mail: bhpr@rheumatology.org.uk
Website: www.rheumatology.org.uk/BHPR

Rheumatology Nursing Forum
RCN Headquarters
Royal College of Nursing
20 Cavendish Square
London, England
WIM ODB
Telephone: 01782-642551
Website: www.rcn.org.uk/services/profess/forums/clinical.htm

UNITED STATES AND CANADA

Association of Rheumatology Health Professionals
A Division of the American College of Rheumatology
The ARHP is responsible for *Arthritis Care and Research,* a scientific journal published bimonthly for arthritis health professionals, as well as *Clinical Care in the Rheumatic Diseases,* an authoritative clinical reference text for physicians and health professionals. ARHP has developed two patient education brochures, briefings on the roles of the various professions within the rheumatology management team, and standards of practice for occupational therapy, physical therapy, social work, and nursing.

1800 Century Place, Suite 250
Atlanta, GA
30345
USA
Telephone: (404) 633-3777
Fax: (404) 633-1870
E-mail: arhp@rheumatology.org
Website: www.rheumatology.org/arhp

MIND-BODY CONNECTION

Books

A Path with Heart, by J. Kornfield. New York: Bantam Books, 1993. ISBN 0553372114

Full Catastrophe Living: Using the Wisdom of Your Body and Mind to Face Stress, Pain, and Illness, by Jon Kabat-Zinn. New York: Dell Publishing, 1990. ISBN 0-3853-03122

Handbook of Coping: Theory, Research, Applications, by M. Zeidner and N. S. Endler (eds.). New York: Wiley, 1996. ISBN 0471599468

Healing and the Mind, by Bill Moyers. New York: Doubleday, 1993. (There is also a "Healing and the Mind" documentary video series—check your local library.) ISBN 0385476876

Love and Survival, by D. Ornish. New York: Harper Collins, 1998. ISBN 0060172134

Mind Body Medicine: How to Use Your Mind for Better Health by D. Goleman and J. Gurin J. (eds.). Yonkers, New York: Consumer Reports Books, 1993. ISBN 0890438404

Molecules of Emotion: the Science Behind Mind-Body Medicine by C. Pert. New York: Scribner, 1997. ISBN 0-6848-3187-2

Molecules of Emotion: Why You Feel The Way You Feel by C. Pert and D. Chopra. Simon and Schuster, 1997.

Opening Up: The Healing Power of Confiding in Others, by J. W. Pennebaker. New York: William Morrow and Company, Inc, 1990.

Opening Up: The Healing Power of Expressing Emotions by J. W. Pennebaker. New York: Guilford Publications, 1997. ISBN 1572302380

Programs and Services

ARTHRITIS SELF-MANAGEMENT PROGRAM (ASMP)

This health promotion program is taught over a six-week period, in weekly two-hour sessions. Classes are led by trained volunteers, who in many cases have arthritis themselves. In a supportive group environment, participants learn skills for managing pain, dealing with stress and depression, problem solving, working with their health care team, and much more. For the small cost of attending, you also get a copy of "The Arthritis Helpbook" by Dr. James Fries and Dr. Kate Lorig. ASMP is available in many communities: Call your local arthritis organization for details.

United States of America

The Arthritis Foundation
P.O. Box 7669
Atlanta, GA
30357-0669
Telephone: (404) 872-7100
E-mail: help@arthritis.org
Website: www.arthritis.org

Canada

The Arthritis Society
393 University Avenue, Suite 1700
Toronto, Ontario
M5G 1E6
Telephone: (416) 979-7228
Toll free information and support: 1-800-321-1433
E-mail:info@arthritis.ca
Website: http://www.arthritis.ca

United Kingdom

In the United Kingdom, a program similar to ASMP is offered, known as
"Arthritis Challenge."
Arthritis Care
18 Stephenson Way
London, NW1 2HD
Telephone: 020 7380 6500
Fax: 020 7380 6505
Website: www.arthritis.bocc.net

CONNECT AND CONTROL

World Wide Web

This fifty-two-week online program supports you in setting up and following through on a personalized self-management program. It includes
information, guidance, support, goal setting, and a personal health diary.
For more information, visit www.arthritis.org and click on "Connect and
Control."

EXERCISE CLASSES

As discussed in Chapter 5, exercise (including both rehabilitative and recreational exercise) is an essential part of your PLAN TO WIN. For information
on land- and water-based arthritis exercise programs in your area, contact:

United States of America

The Arthritis Foundation
P.O. Box 7669
Atlanta, GA
30357-0669
USA
Toll free: 1-800-283-7800
E-mail: help@arthritis.org
Website: www.arthritis.org

Canada

The Arthritis Society
393 University Avenue, Suite 1700
Toronto, Ontario M5G 1E6
416-979-7228
Toll free: 1-800-321-1433.
E-mail: info@arthritis.ca
Website: http://www.arthritis.ca
Other exercise and self management programs might be available in your
community—contact your local arthritis organization or community/
recreation center.

Medical Publications

Rheumatology Text Books

Arthritis and Allied Conditions—A Textbook of Rheumatology, by W. J. Koopman, 14th ed. Philadelphia: Lippincott Williams & Wilkins, 2001. ISBN 0781722403

Clinical Care in the Rheumatic Diseases, by S. T. Wegener, et al. Atlanta, GA: American College of Rheumatology, 1996. ISBN 0965431606

Kelley's Textbook of Rheumatology, E. D. Harris, Jr., S. Ruddy, and C. B. Sledge (eds.). Philadelphia: W. B. Saunders, 6th ed., 2001. ISBN 0721680089

Nutrition and Rheumatic Diseases, by R. S. Panush, Rheumatic Disease Clinics of North America, Vol. 17, No. 2. 1991.

Oxford Textbook of Rheumatology, by P. J. Maddison, D. A. Isenberg, P. Woo, and D. N. Glas (eds.). Second Edition. 2 vol. set. New York: Oxford University Press, 1998. ISBN 0192626973

Primer on the Rheumatic Diseases, J. H. Klippel (ed.). 11th ed. Atlanta, GA: Arthritis Foundation, 1998. ISBN 0912423161

Rheumatoid Arthritis, by E. D. Harris, Jr. Philadelphia: W. B. Saunders, 1997. ISBN 0721652492

Rheumatoid Arthritis: Frontiers in Pathogenesis and Treatment, by G. S. Firestein (ed.). New York: Oxford University Press, 2000. ISBN 0192629727

Rheumatology, J. H. Klippel and P. A. Dieppe (eds). 2nd ed. 2 vols. London: Mosby International, 1998. ISBN 0723424055

Treatment of the Rheumatic Diseases: Companion to the Textbook of Rheumatology, Michael H. Weisman and Michael E. Weinblatt (ed.). Philadelphia: W. B. Saunders, 1995. ISBN 0721653820

Rheumatology Journals

Almost every day, somewhere in the world a new study is being published on RA. These studies are collected in scientific journals, written by and for medical professionals, but they are also good places for people with RA to keep abreast of current knowledge. Even if you have no medical background, it is possible to understand enough of what's written (particularly in the "abstracts," which are short summaries of the research) to enable you to have more informed conversations about current practice with your health care team members.

Also, if you live in a smaller community where it's not possible to find rheumatologists, physiotherapists, and occupational therapists who are RA specialists, these journals may serve as useful as reference material for you to recommend or pass along to your health care team members.

Bound copies of these journals are available at libraries, and of course, are also available by paid subscription (which is generally quite expensive). However, many do offer a free table of contents e-mail service (they will e-mail the full list of articles to you each time a new volume of the journal is published, often with links to the full articles.) This is an easy, inexpensive way to keep in touch with current research; to subscribe, simply visit the journal's website and, if the service is offered, fill in the online order form.

Annals of the Rheumatic Diseases
Features original work in all aspects of rheumatology and connective tissue disorders. Publishes clinical, epidemiological, and laboratory reports, hypothesis articles, and clinical teaching. Monthly.

BMJ Publishing Group
BMA House
Tavistock Square
London WC1H 9JR
United Kingdom
Telephone: 020 7383 6270
Fax: 020 7383 6402
E-mail: subscriptions@bmjgroup.com
Website: ard.bmjjournals.com

Arthritis Care and Research
The official journal of the American College of Rheumatology and the Association of Rheumatology Health Professionals. Publishes articles concerning clinical problems and research, as well as economic, educational, and social issues. Six issues per year.

John Wiley & Sons, Inc.
605 Third Avenue
New York, NY
10158
USA
Telephone: (212) 850-6645
E-mail: subinfo@wiley.com
Website: www.interscience.wiley.com

Arthritis and Rheumatism
An official journal of the American College of Rheumatology. Covers all aspects of inflammatory disease.

John Wiley & Sons, Inc.
605 Third Avenue
New York, NY
10158
USA
Telephone: 1-800-825-7550 (in USA), (212) 850-6645 (outside USA)
Website: www.interscience.wiley.com

Best Practice & Research Clinical Rheumatology
Each topic-based issue contains information on the latest best practice and clinical evidence in rheumatology. Published five times a year.

Harcourt Publishers
Foots Cray High Street
Sidcup
Kent
DA14 5HP
United Kingdom
Telephone: 020 8308 5700
Fax: 020 8308 5702
E-mail: cservice@harcourt.com
Website: www.harcourt-international.com

Clinical and Experimental Rheumatology
A forum on international advances in rheumatology. Abstracts can be read online at http://www.clinexprheumatol.org.

via Santa Maria 31
56126 Pisa, Italy
FAX: 050 50.22.99

Clinical Rheumatology
An international journal devoted to original clinical investigation and research in rheumatology, with emphasis on clinical aspects at the postgraduate level. Six issues per year. Free table of contents e-mail service.

Springer-Verlag London Limited
Sweetapple House
Catteshall Road
Godalming
Surrey GU7 3DJ
United Kingdom
Telephone: 01483 418822
Fax: 01483 415151
E-mail: postmaster@svl.co.uk
Website: http://link.springer.de/link/service/journals/10067/index.htm

Current Opinion in Rheumatology
Publishes the views of experts on current advances in rheumatology.

Lippincott Williams & Wilkins, Ltd.
530 Walnut Street
Philadelphia, PA 19106
USA
Telephone: (215) 521-8300
Fax: (215) 521-8902
Website: www.co-rheumatology.com

Journal of Rheumatology
Clinical subjects, original research, symposia on topics of interest and new developments in the field of rheumatology. Monthly. You can read the current issue or search the archives by topic online at: http://www.jrheum.com/current.html

920 Yonge St., Ste. 115,
Toronto, ON M4W 3C7
Canada
Telephone: (416) 967-5155
Fax: (416) 967-7556
Website: www.jrheum.com

Rheumatology
Rheumatology (formerly the British Journal of Rheumatology) publishes original clinical, laboratory, and therapeutic research, as well as papers on rehabilitation. In addition to many full length original research papers, each issue includes editorials, regular scientific reviews, clinical grand rounds, preliminary and brief papers, viewpoints, book reviews, and a lively correspondence section. Read the table of contents and abstracts of the current edition online at: http://rheumatology.oupjournals.org or subscribe to the free table of contents e-mail service. Only paid subscribers can read the current or archived articles online.

In USA and Canada:
Oxford University Press
Journals Marketing
2001 Evans Rd.
Cary, NC 27513
USA
Telephone: (919) 677-0977
Toll free: 1-800-852-7323
Email: jnlorders@oup-usa.org
Website: http://rheumatology.oupjournals.org

Elsewhere:
Journals Marketing,
Oxford University Press,
Great Clarendon Street,
Oxford OX2 6DP
United Kingdom

Seminars in Arthritis and Rheumatism

Seminars in Arthritis and Rheumatism provides a broad interpretation of the field, including aspects of general medicine and orthopedics. Each bimonthly issue presents comprehensive review articles focusing on topics in rheumatology. Available to order and view online.

Harcourt Health Services
Subscription Customer Service
6277 Sea Harbor Drive
Orlando, FL 32887-4800
USA
Telephone (USA): 1-800-654-2452, International: (407) 345-4066
Fax: (407) 363-9661
E-mail: hhspcs@harcourt.com
Website: www.harcourthealth.com/fcgi-bin/displaypage.pl?isbn=00490172

Scandinavian Journal of Rheumatology

The journal is an international scientific journal covering clinical and experimental aspects of rheumatic diseases.

Taylor and Francis Group
11 New Fetter Lane
London EC4P 4EE
UK
Tel: 0 20 7583 9855
Fax: 0 20 7842 2298
E-mail: journals.orders@tandf.co.uk
Website: www.tandf.co.uk/journals/frameloader.html?
http://www.tandf.co.uk/journals/tfs/03009742.html

The Medical Letter

A nonprofit peer-reviewed publication with unbiased, in-depth information and studies on medications. Available to order and view online.

The Medical Letter, Inc.
1000 Main Street
New Rochelle, NY
10801
USA
Telephone: 1-800-211-2769 or (914) 235-0500
Fax: (914) 632-1733
E-mail: custserv@themedicalletter.org
Website: www.medicalletter.com

Major Medical Journals

Most of the important, groundbreaking studies in RA and arthritis in general appear first in the following major medical journals:

New England Journal of Medicine
Massachusetts Medical Society
10 Shattuck Street
Boston, MA
02115-6094
USA
Telephone: (617) 734-9800
Fax: (617) 739-9864
Website: www.nejm.org

The Lancet
84 Theobald's Road
London, WC1X 8RR
UK
Fax: 020 7611 4479
Website: www.thelancet.com/journal
Journal of the American Medical Association
Subscriber Services Center
American Medical Association
P.O. Box 10946
Chicago, IL 60610-0946
USA
Telephone: 1-800-262-2350 or (312) 670-7827
E-mail: ama-subs@ama-assn.org
Website: http://jama.ama-assn.org

British Medical Journal
BMJ Publishing Group
P.O. Box 299
London WC1H 9TD

UK
Fax: 0 + 44 (0)20 383 6455
E-mail: subscriptions@bmjgroup.com
Website: www.bmj.com

In the USA:
BMJ Publishing Group
P.O. Box 590A
Kennebunkport, ME 04046
USA
Telephone 1-800-236-6265
E-mail: bjpaige@cybertours.com

Annals of Internal Medicine
American Society of Internal Medicine
190 N. Independence Mall
West Philadelphia, PA 19106-1572
USA
Telephone: 1-800-523-1546 extension 2600 or (215) 351-2600
Website: www.annals.org

American Journal of Medicine
Excerpta Medica, Inc.
P.O. Box 7247-7197
Philadelphia, PA 19170-7197
USA
Telephone: from within the United States: (800) 606-0023
          from outside the United States: (609) 786-0841
Fax: (609) 786-7032
E-mail: ajm@medicine.ucsf.edu
Website: www.amjmed.org

Online Databases
United States National Library of Medicine
"The world's largest medical library and the creator of Medline [on online medical library search service]."

www.nlm.nih.gov

Medscape
Access to Medline and other databases. Includes up-to-date medical news, reference service, and member information. Free registration.

www.medscape.com

Combined Health Information Database
This database produced by health-related agencies of the U.S.A. Federal Government. It provides titles, abstracts, and lists a wealth of health promotion and education materials and program descriptions that are not indexed elsewhere.

http://chid.aerie.com

www.medlib.iupui.edu
This resource is a collaborative effort between the Ruth Lilly Medical Library, and the HealthWeb project. HealthWeb is a cooperative project of the health sciences libraries of the Committee on Institutional Cooperation.

CLINICAL TRIALS

http://www.cc.nih.gov/ccc/prpl/
You can search the National Institutes of Health's (NIH) Patient Recruitment and Public Liaison Office's web page for RA-related, NIH-funded clinical trials in the United States. Phone numbers and e-mail links are provided if you wish to inquire further about specific studies.

http://clinicaltrails.gov/ct/gui/c/r
This page is part of the National Library of Medicine's website. It lists clinical trials in the United States funded by the NIH (there is some duplication with those found on the above listed site), and others. Information is well presented and quite comprehensive.

http://www.arthritis.ca/clinicaltrials
This site lists clinical trials (by arthritis type) being conducted in Canada and provides a clear description of the "ins and outs" of participating in clinical trials, such as: what is a clinical trial; making the decision to participate; glossary of clinical trial terms; and other topics.

CHAPTER 2

1. Arnett F. C., Edworthy S. M., Bloch D. A., et al., "The American Rheumatism Association 1987 revised criteria for the classification of rheumatoid arthritis." *Arthritis and Rheumatism.* 31, pp. 315–324, 1988.

CHAPTER 3

1. Lorig, K., Holman, H., Sobel, D., Laurent, D., Gonzalez, V., and Minor, M., *Living a Healthy Life with Chronic Conditions: Self Management of Heart Disease, Arthritis, Diabetes, Asthma, Bronchitis, Emphysema & Others.* Palo Alto: Bull Publishing Company, pp. 11-19, 1994.

2   Wallace, J., *Arthritis Relief: A Take-Charge Plan of Positive Nutrition, Gentle Exercise, Relaxation, Medical Care, and Everyday Coping Tips.* PA: Rodale Books, p. 45, 1989.

3. Holman, H., and Lorig, K., "Patient Education: Essential to Good Healthcare for Patients with Chronic Arthritis." *Arthritis and Rheumatism.* Aug. 40(8), pp. 1371-1373, 1997.

4. Adapted from Arthritis Foundation, *Your Personal Guide,* 1998.

5. Arthritis Foundation, p. 33, 1988.

6. Sobel, D., and Klein, A. C., *Arthritis: What Works.* New York: St. Martin's Press, pp. 21-25, 1989.

7. Orlock, C., "The Power of Partnership." *Arthritis Today.* Nov/Dec., p. 28, 1993.

8. Badley, E. M., Rasooly, I., and Webster, G. K., "Relative importance of musculoskeletal disorders as a cause of chronic health problems, dis-

ability and health utilization: Findings from the 1990 Ontario Health Survey." *Journal of Rheumatology.* 21, pp. 505–514, 1994.

9. Reynolds, D. L., Chambers, L. W., Badley, E. M., Bennett, K. J., Goldsmith, C. H., Jamieson, E., Torrance, G. W., and Tugwell, P., "Physical disability among Canadians reporting musculoskeletal diseases." *Journal of Rheumatology.* 19, pp. 1020–1030, 1992.

10. Wallace, p. 240, 1989.

11. From an interview with Greg Taylor, social worker with The Arthritis Society of Canada, BC and Yukon Division, Spring 1999.

12. Sobel and Klein, pp. 169–170, 1989.

13. Ibid., pp. 172–173.

14. Kane J., *Be Sick Well.* Oakland: New Harbinger Publications, p. 79, 1991.

15. McCall T., "The Right Stuff." *Arthritis Today.* July/Aug, pp. 21-22, 1996.

16. Arthritis Foundation, p. 46, 1998.

17. Arthritis Foundation, p. 7, 1998.

18. Bradley, L. A., "Adherence with treatment regimens among rheumatoid arthritis patients: Current status and future directions." *Arthritis Care.* 2, pp. 533–539, 1989.

19. Ferguson, K. and Gold, G. G., "Family support, health, belief and therapeutic compliance in patients with RA." *Patient Counsel Health Education.* 1, pp. 101-105, 1979.

CHAPTER 4

1. Scott, D. L. et al., "Long-term outcome of treating rheumatoid arthritis: results after 20 years." *The Lancet.* 1, pp. 1108–1111, 1987.

2. Pincus, T., and Callahan, L. F., "Remodeling the pyramid or remodeling the paradigms concerning rheumatoid arthritis—lessons from Hodgkin's disease and coronary artery disease." *Journal of Rheumatology.* 17, pp. 1582–1585, 1990.

3. Fuchs, H. A., Kaye, J. J., Callahan, L. F., and Pincus, T., "Evidence of significant radiographic damage in rheumatoid arthritis within the first two years of disease." *Journal of Rheumatology.* 16, pp. 585–591, 1989.

4. Egmose, C., Lund, B., Borg, G., Pettersson, H., Berg, E., Brodin, U., and Trang, L., "Patients with rheumatoid arthritis benefit from early 2nd line therapy: 5–year follow-up of a prospective double blind placebo controlled study. *Journal of Rheumatology.* 22, pp. 2208–2213, 1995.

5. Tsakonas, E., Fitzgerald, A. A., Fitzcharles, M.A., Cividino, A., Thorne, J. C., and Esdaile, J. M., "Consequences of delayed therapy with second-line agents in rheumatoid arthritis (HERA) study." *Journal of Rheumatology.* 27(3), pp. 623–629, 2000.

6. Fries JF, Williams CA, Morfeld D. Singh G, Sibley J. Reduction in long-term disability in patients with rheumatoid arthritis by disease-modi-

fying antirheumatic drug-based treatment strategies. *Arthritis and Rheumatism* 1996; 39: 616–622.

7. Neville, C., Fortin, P. R., Fitzcharles, M., Baron, M., Abrahamowitz, M., Du Berger, R., et al. "The Needs of Patients with Arthritis: The Patient's Perspective." *Arthritis Care and Research.* pp. 85–95, 1999.

8. Thomason, T. E., McCune, J. S., Bernard, S. A., Winer, E. P., Tremont, S., and Lindley, C. M., "Cancer pain survey: patient-centred issues in control." *Journal of Pain Symptom Management.* 15(5), pp. 275–84, 1998.

9. Stross, J. K., "Relationships between knowledge and experience in the use of disease-modifying antirheumatic agents: A study of primary care practitioners." *Journal of the American Medical Association.* 262(19): pp. 2721-2723, 1989.

10. Bradley, L. A., "Adherence with treatment regimens among rheumatoid arthritis patients: Current status and future directions." *Arthritis Care and Research.* 2 (Supplement), S33–S39, 1989.

11. Ferguson, K., and Bold G. G., "Family support, health, belief and therapeutic compliance in patients with rheumatoid arthritis." *Patient Counselling and Health Education.* 1, pp. 101-105, 1979.

12. Lorish, C. D., Richards, B., and Brown, S., Jr., "Perspective of the patient with rheumatoid arthritis on issues related to missed medication." *Arthritis Care and Research.* 3, pp. 78–84, 1990.

13. Feinberg, J., "The effect of patient-practitioner interaction on compliance: A review of the literature and application in rheumatoid arthritis." *Patient Education and Counselling.* 11, pp. 171-187, 1988.

14. Sleath, B., Roter, D., Chewning, B., and Svarstad, B., "Asking questions about medications: Analysis of physician-patient interactions and physician perceptions." *Medical Care.* 37(11), pp. 1169–1173, 1999.

15. Klippel, J. H. et al., *Primer on the rheumatic diseases.* 11th ed. Atlanta, GA: Arthritis Foundation, p. 169, 1997.

16. Tramer, M. R., Moore, R. A., Reynolds, D. J., and McQuay, H. J., "Quantitative estimation of rare adverse events which follow a biological progression: a new model applied to chronic NSAID use." *Pain.* 85(1-2), pp. 169–182, 2000.

17. Lipsky, P. E., et al., "Analysis of the effect of COX-2 specific inhibitors and recommendations for their use in clinical practice." (Editorial). *Journal of Rheumatology.* 27(6), pp. 1338–1340, 2000.

18. Singh, G., Ramey, D. R., Morfeld, D., Shi, H., Hartoum, H. T., and Fries, J. F., "Gastrointestinal tract complications of nonsteroidal anti-inflammatory drug treatment in rheumatoid arthritis. A prospective observational cohort study." *Archives of Internal Medicine.* 156 (14), pp. 1530–1536, 1996.

CHAPTER 5

1. Ekblom, B., Lovgren, O., Alderin, M., Friedstrom, M., and Satterstrom, G., "Effect of short-term physical training on patients with rheumatoid arthritis: A six-month follow-up study." *Scandinavian Journal of Rheumatology.* 4, pp. 80–86, 1975.

2. Nordemar, R., Ekblom, B., Zachrisson, L., and Lundquist, K., "Physical training in rheumatoid arthritis: A controlled long-term study. *Scandinavian Journal of Rheumatology.* 10, pp. 17–23, 1981.

3. Harkom, T. M., Lampman, R. M., Banwell, B. F., and Castor, C. W., "Therapeutic value of graded aerobic exercise training in rheumatoid arthritis." *Arthritis and Rheumatism.* 28, pp. 32–39, 1985.

4. Semble, E. L., Loeser, R. F., and Wise, C. M., "Therapeutic exercise for rheumatoid arthritis and osteoarthritis." *Seminars in Arthritis and Rheumatism.* 20, pp. 32–40, 1990.

5. Harkom, Lampman, Banwell, and Castor, 1985.

6. Byers, P. H., "Effect of exercise on morning stiffness and mobility in patients with rheumatoid arthritis." *Research in Nursing and Health.* 8, pp. 275–281, 1985.

CHAPTER 6

1. Helliwell, M., Coombes, E. J., Moodly, B. J., et al., "Nutritional status in patients with rheumatoid arthritis." *Annals of Rheumatic Disease.* 43, p. 386–390, 1987.

2. Kremer, J. M., "Nutrition and Rheumatic Diseases." In Harris, E. D. Jr., Ruddy, S., and Sledge, C. B., *Kelley's Textbook of Rheumatology, 6th Edition, Vol. 1.* Philadelphia, W. B. Saunders, p. 713, 2000.

3. Lau, C. S., Morley, K. D., and Belch, J. J. "Effects of fish oil supplementation on non-steroidal anti-inflammatory drug requirement in patients with mild rheumatoid arthritis—a double-blind placebo controlled study." *British Journal of Rheumatology.* 32, pp. 982–989, 1993.

4. Kremer, J. M., Lawrence, D. A., Petrillo, G. F., Litts, L. L., Mullaly, P. M., Rynes, R. I, Stocker, R. P., Parhami, N., Greenstein, H. S., Fuchs, B. R. et al. "Effects of high-dose fish oil on rheumatoid arthritis after stopping nonsterioidal antiinflammatory drugs. Clinical and immune correlates." *Arthritis and Rheumatism.* 38(8), pp. 1107–1114, 1995.

5. U.S. Department of Agriculture, U.S. Department of Health and Human Services, *Nutrition and Your Health: Dietary Guidelines for Americans.* Fifth edition, Washington D.C. 2000.

6. Palmblad, J., Hafstrom, I., and Ringertz, B., "Antirheumatic effects of fasting." *Rheumatic Disease Clinics of North America.* 17, p. 351-362, 1991.

7. Skoldstam, L., and Magnusson, K. E., "Fasting, intestinal permeability, and rheumatoid arthritis." *Rheumatic Disease Clinics of North America.* 17(2), pp. 363–371, 1991.

8. Eisenberg, D. M., Kessler, R. C., Roster, C., et al., "Unconventional medicine in the United States." *New England Journal of Medicine.* 328, pp. 246–252, 1993.

9. Tzu Chi Institute for Complementary and Alternative Medicine, www.tci.bc.ca. Vancouver, 2001.

10. Eisenberg, D. M., Roger, B. D, Ettner, S. L., Appel, S., Wilkey, S., Van Rompay, M., and Kessler, R. C., "Trends in alternative medicine use in the United States, 1990–1997: Results of a Follow-up National Survey." *Journal of the American Medical Association.* 280, pp. 1569–1575, 1998.

11. Ramsay, C., Walker, M., and Alexander J., "Alternative medicine in Canada: Use and public attitudes." Fraser Institute. March, 1999.

12. Rasmussen, N. K., and Morgall, J. M., "The use of alternative treatments in the Danish adult population." *Complementary Medicine Research.* 4:156–22, 1990.

13. Vaskilampi, T., Merilainen, P., Sinkkonen, S., et al., "The use of alternative treatments in the Finnish adult population." In Lewith G. T., and Aldridge D., (eds.), *Clinical Research Methodology for Complementary Therapies.* London: Hodder & Stoughton, pp. 204–229, 1993.

14. MacLennan, H. H., Wilson, D. H., and Taylor, W. W., "Prevalence and cost of alternative medicine in Australia." *The Lancet.* 347, pp. 569–573, 1996.

15. Rao, J. K., Mihaliak, K., Kroenke, K., Bradley, J., Tierney, W. M., and Weinberger, M., "Use of Complementary Therapies for Arthritis among Patients of Rheumatologists." *Annals of Internal Medicine.* 131, pp. 409–416, 1999.

16. Morgan, S. L., Baggott, J. E., Vaughn, W. H., et al., "Supplementation with folic acid during methotrexate therapy for rheumatoid arthritis: A double-blind placebo-controlled trial." *Annals of Internal Medicine.* 121, p. 833–841, 1994.

17. Shiroky, J. B., Nevill, C., Esdaile, J. M., et al., "Low-dose methotrexate with leucovorin (folinic acid) in the management of rheumatoid arthritis. Results of a randomized, double-blind, placebo-controlled trial." *Arthritis and Rheumatism.* 36, p. 795–803, 1993.

18. Monkman, D. and Dingwell, G., "Watching for Red Flags: when should you worry about your choices?" Vancouver, BC: Tzu Chi Institute, 2000.

CHAPTER 7

1. Lazar, J. S., "Mind-body medicine in primary care: Implications and applications." *Primary Care.* 23(1), pp. 169–182, 1996.

2. Goleman, D., and Gurin, J. (eds.), *Mind Body Medicine: How to Use Your Mind for Better Health.* New York: Consumer Reports Books, 1993.

3. Lazar, 1996.

4. Goleman and Gurin, 1993.

5. Lazar, 1996.

6. Anderson, K. O., Bradley, L. A., Young, L. D., McDaniel, L. K., and Wise, C. M., "Rheumatoid arthritis: Review of psychological factors related to etiology, effects, and treatment." *Psychological Bulletin.* 98(2), pp. 358–387, 1985.

7. Lazar, 1996.

8. Lazar, 1996.

9. Lazar, 1996.

10. Moran, M.G., "Pulmonary and rheumatologic diseases." In A. Stoudemire (ed.), *Psychological Factors Affecting Medical Conditions.* Washington, DC: American Psychiatric Press, Inc., pp. 141-158, 1995.

11. Moran, 1995.

12. Aviäna-Zubieta, J.A., Pâaez, F., and Galindo-Rodriguez, G., "Rheumatic manifestations of neurologic and psychiatric diseases." *Current Opinion in Rheumatology.* 9(1), pp. 51-5, 1997.

13. Young, L. D., "Psychological factors in rheumatoid arthritis." *Journal of Consulting and Clinical Psychology.* 60(4), pp. 619–627, 1990.

14. Anderson, K. O., Bradley, L. A., Young, L. D., McDaniel, L. K., and Wise, C. M., "Rheumatoid arthritis: Review of psychological factors related to etiology, effects, and treatment." *Psychological Bulletin.* 98(2), pp. 358–387, 1985.

15. Astin, J. A., Shapiro, S. L., Lee, R. A., and Shapiro, D. H., "The construct of control in mind-body medicine: Implications for healthcare." *Alternative Therapies in Health and Medicine.* 5(2), pp. 42–47, 1999.

16. Huyser, B. A., and Parker, J. C., "Negative affect and pain in arthritis." *Rheumatic Diseases Clinics of North America.* 25(1), pp. 105–21, 1998.

17. Young, 1990.

18. Kubler-Ross, E., *On Death and Dying.* New York: Macmilllan, 1969.

19. Rogers, M.P., "Rheumatoid arthritis: Psychiatric aspects and use of psychotropics." *Psychosomatics,* 26(12), pp. 915–925 1985.

20. Halliday, J. L., "Psychological aspects of rheumatoid arthritis." *Proceedings of the Royal Society of Medicine.* 35, pp. 455–457, 1942.

21. Creed, F., and Ash, G., "Depression in rheumatoid arthritis: Aetiology and treatment." *International Review of Psychiatry,* 4(1), pp. 23–33. 1992.

22. Young, 1990.

23. Pincus, T., Griffith, J., Pearce, S., and Isenberg, D. "Prevalence of self-reported depression in patients with rheumatoid arthritis." *British Journal of Rheumatology,* 35(9), pp. 879–83 1996.

24. Callahan, L. F., and Blalock, S. J., "Behavioral and social research in rheumatology." *Current Opinion in Rheumatology.* 9(2), pp. 126–132, 1997.

25. Young, 1990.

26. Katon, W., and Sullivan, M. D., "Depression and chronic medical illness," *Journal of Clinical Psychiatry.* 51(6, Suppl.), pp. 3–11, 1990.
27. Callahan and Blalock, 1997.
28. Moldofsky, H., and Rothman, A. I., "Personality, disease parameters and medication in rheumatoid arthritis." *Journal of Chronic Diseases.* 24(6), pp. 363–372, 1971.
29. Robinson, H., Kirk, R. F. and Frye, R. L., "A psychological study of rheumatoid arthritis and selected controls." *Journal of Chronic Diseases.* 23, pp. 791-801, 1971.
30. Pincus, T., Griffith, J., Pearce, S., and Isenberg, D., 1996.
31. Creed and Ash, 1992.
32. Creed and Ash, 1992.
33. Katon and Sullivan, 1990.
34. Creed and Ash, 1992.
35. Wallace, D. J., "Does stress or trauma cause or aggravate rheumatic disease?" *Bailliere's Clinical Rheumatology.* 8(1), pp. 149–159, 1994.
36. Katon and Sullivan, 1990.
37. Hayes, A. "Psychiatric nursing: What does biology have to do with it?" *Archives of Psychiatric Nursing.* 9(4), pp. 216–224, 1995.
38. Pincus, Griffith, Pearce, and Isenberg, 1996.
39. Creed and Ash, 1992.
40. Greer, S., and Morris, T., "Psychological attributes of women who develop breast cancer." *Journal of Psychosomatic Research.* 19, pp. 147–153, 1975.
41. Smyth, J. M., Stone, A. A., Hurewitz, A., and Kaell, A., "Effects of writing about stressful experiences on symptom reduction in patients with asthma or rheumatoid arthritis: A randomized trial." *Journal of the American Medical Association.* 218(14), pp. 1304–1309, 1999.
42. McFarlane, A. C., Kalucy, R. S., and Brooks, P. M., "Psychological predictors of disease course in rheumatoid arthritis." *Journal of Psychosomatic Research.* 31(6), pp. 757–764, 1987.
43. Nakajima, A., Hirai, H., and Yoshino, S. "Reassessment of mirthful laughter in rheumatoid arthritis." *Journal of Rheumatology.* 26(2), pp. 512–513, 1999.
44. Huyser, B. A., and Parker, J. C., "Negative affect and pain in arthritis." *Rheumatic Diseases Clinics of North America.* 25(1), pp. 105–121, 1998.
45. Goleman and Gurin, 1993.
46. McFarlane, Kalucy, and Brooks, 1987.
47. Hayes, 1995.
48. Goleman and Gurin, 1993.
49. Goleman and Gurin, 1993.
50. Goleman and Gurin, 1993.
51. Greer, 1991.

52. Huyser and Parker, 1998.

53. Astin, Shapiro, S. L., Lee, and Shapiro, D. H., 1999.

54. Smith, T. W., Peck, J. R., Milano, R. A., and Ward, J. R., "Cognitive distortion in rheumatoid arthritis: Relation to depression and disability." *Journal of Consulting and Clinical Psychology.* 56, pp. 412–416, 1998.

55. Persson, L. O., Berglund, K., and Sahlberg, D., "Psychological factors in chronic rheumatic diseases—a review: The case of rheumatoid arthritis, current research and some problems." *Scandinavian Journal of Rheumatology.* 28(3), pp. 137–144, 1999.

56. Callahan, L. F., and Pincus, T., "The sense of coherence scale in patients with rheumatoid arthritis." *Arthritis Care and Research.* 8(1), pp. 28–35, 1995.

57. Schnyder, U., Buechi, Moergeli, H., Sensky, T., and Klaghofer, R., "Sense of coherence—a mediator between disability and handicap?" *Psychotherapy and Psychosomatics.* 68(2), pp. 102–110, 1999.

58. Beuchi, S., Sensky, T., Allard, S., Stoll, T., Schnyder, U., Klaghofer, R., and Buddeberg, C., "Sense of coherence—a protective factor for depression in rheumatoid arthritis." *Journal of Rheumatology.* 25(5), pp. 869–875, 1998.

59. Persson, Berglund, and Sahlberg, 1999.

60. Goleman and Gurin, 1993.

61. Zeidner, M., and Endler, N. S. (eds.), *Handbook of Coping: Theory, Research, Applications.* New York: Wiley, 1996.

62. Zautra, A. J., and Manne, S. L., "Coping with rheumatoid arthritis: A review of a decade of research." *Annals of Behavioral Medicine.* 14(1), pp. 31-39, 1992.

63. Zeidner and Endler, 1996.

64. Astin, Shapiro S. L., Lee, and Shapiro, D. H., 1999.

65. Astin, Shapiro S. L., Lee, and Shapiro, D. H., 1999.

66. Young, 1990.

67. Zautra and Manne, 1992.

68. Astin, Shapiro, S. L., Lee, and Shapiro, D. H., 1999.

69. Persson, Berglund, and Sahlberg, 1999.

70. Astin, Shapiro, S. L., Lee, and Shapiro, D. H., 1999.

71. Persson, Berglund, and Sahlberg, 1999.

72. Astin, Shapiro, S. L., Lee, and Shapiro, D. H., 1999.

73. Astin, Shapiro, S. L., Lee, and Shapiro, D. H., 1999.

74. Goleman and Gurin, 1993.

75. O'Leary, A., Shoor, S., Loring, K., and Holman, H. R., "A cognitive behavioral treatment for rheumatoid arthritis," *Health Psychology.* 7, pp. 527–544, 1988.

76. Goleman and Gurin, 1993.

77. Hoffman, J. W., Benson, H., Arns, P. A., et al., "Reduced sympathetic nervous system responsivity associated with the relaxation response," *Science.* 215, pp. 190–192, 1982.

78. Kabat-Zinn, J., Lipworth, L., Burney, R., et al., "Four year follow-up of a meditation-based program for the self-regulation of chronic pain: Treatment outcomes and compliance." *Clinical Journal of Pain.* 2, pp. 159–173,1986.

79. Kaplan, K. H., Goldenberg, D. L., and Galvin-Nadeau, M., "The impact of a meditation-based stress-reduction program on fibromyalgia." *General Hospital Psychiatry.* 15, pp. 284–289, 1993.

80. Denver, D. R., Laveault, D., Girard, F., Lacourciere, Y., Latulippe, L., Grove, R. N., Preve, M., and Doiron, N., "Behavioral medicine: Biobehavioral effects of short-term thermal biofeedback and relaxation in rheumatoid arthritis patients," *Biofeedback and Self-Regulation.* 4, pp. 245–246, 1979.

81. Achterberg, J., McGraw, P., and Lawlis, G. F., "Rheumatoid arthritis: A study of relaxation and temperature biofeedback training as an adjunctive therapy," *Biofeedback and Self-Regulation.* 6, pp. 207–223, 1981.

82. Gruber, B. L., Hall, N. R. Hersh, S. P., et al., "Immune system and psychological changes in metstatic cancer patients using relaxation and guided imagery: A pilot study." *Scandinavian Journal of Behavior Therapy.* 17, pp. 25–45, 1988.

83. Schnyder, U., Buechi, Moergeli, H., Sensky, T., and Klaghofer, R., 1999.

84. Benson, H., Beary, J. F., and Carol, M. P., "The relaxation response," *Psychiatry.* 37, pp. 37–46, 1974.

85. Callahan and Blalock, 1997.

86. Young, 1990.

87. Callahan and Blalock, 1997.

88. Bradley, L. A., Young, L. D., Anderson, K. O., Turner, R. A., Agudelo, C. A., McDaniel, L. K., Pisko, E. J., Semble, E. L., and Morgan, T. M., "Effects of psychological therapy on pain behavior of rheumatoid arthritis patients: Treatment outcome and six-month follow-up." *Arthritis and Rheumatism.* 30, pp. 1105–1114, 1987.

89. Callahan and Blalock, 1997.

90. Huyser, B., and Parker, J. C., "Stress and rheumatoid arthritis: An integrative review." *Arthritis Care and Research.* 11(2), pp. 135–145, 1998.

91. McCracken, L. M., "Cognitive-behavioral treatment of rheumatoid arthritis: A preliminary review of efficacy and methodology." *Annals of Behavioral Medicine.* 13(2), pp. 57–65, 1991.

92. Young, L. D., 1990.

93. Astin, Shapiro, S. L., Lee, and Shapiro, D. H., 1999.

94. Goleman and Gurin, 1993.

95. Goodenow, C., Reisine, S. T., and Grady, K. E., "Quality of social support and associated social and psychological functioning in women with rheumatoid arthritis." *Health Psychology.* 9, pp. 266–284, 1990.

96. Lanza, A. F., and Revenson, T. A., "Social support interventions for rheumatoid arthritis patients: The cart before the horse?" *Health Education Quarterly.* 20, pp. 97–117, 1993.

97. Baker, G. H. "Invited review: Psychological factors and immunity," *Journal of Psychosomatic Research,* 31(1), pp. 1–10, 1987.

98. Chrisler, J. C., and Parrett, K. L., "Women and autoimmune disorders." In Stanton, A. L. and Gallant, S. J. (eds.), *The Psychology of Women's Health: Progress and Challenges in Research and Application* Washington, DC: American Psychological Association, pp. 171–195, 1995.

99. Goleman and Gurin, 1993.

100. Huyser and Parker, 1998.

101. Anderson, Bradley, Young, McDaniel, and Wise, 1985.

102. Lanza and Revenson, 1993.

103. Goleman and Gurin, 1993.

104. Anderson, Bradley, Young, McDaniel, and Wise, 1985.

105. Horton, J. R., and Mitzdorf, U., "Clinical hypnosis in the treatment of rheumatoid arthritis," *Psychologische Beitraege,* 36(1–2), pp. 205–212, 1994.

106. Goleman and Gurin, 1993.

107. Goleman and Gurin, 1993.

108. Blanchard, E. B., "Behavioral medicine and health psychology." In Bergin, A. E. and Garfield, S.L. (eds.), *Handbook of Psychotherapy and Behavior Change. (4th ed.).* New York: John Wiley and Sons, 1994.

CHAPTER 8

Bibliography

Anderson, K. O., Bradley, L. A., Young, L. D., McDaniel, L. K., and Wise, C. M., "Rheumatoid arthritis: Review of psychological factors related to etiology, effects, and treatment." *Psychological Bulletin,* 98(2), pp. 358–387, 1985.

Baldursson, H., and Brattstrom, J., "Sexual difficulties and total hip replacement in rheumatoid arthritis," *Scandanavian Journal of Rheumatology.* 8, pp. 214–216, 1979.

Barrett, M., "Resources on sexuality and physical disability." In Nagler, M. (ed.), *Perspectives on Disability.* Palo Alto, CA: Health Markets Research, pp. 328–333, 1990.

Becker, J., and Abel, G. G., "Sex and disability: Treatment issues." *Behavioral Medicine Update.* 4(4), pp. 15–20, 1983.

Beckham, J. C., Burker, E. J., Rice, J. R., and Talton, S. L., "Patient predictors of caregiver burden, optimism, and pessimism in rheumatoid arthritis." *Behavioral Medicine,* 30(4), pp. 171–179, 1995.

Blake, D. J., "Sexual aspects of arthritis." In Ahmed, P. I. (ed.), *Coping with Arthritis.* Springfield, IL: Charles C. Thomas, pp. 217–227, 1988.

Blake, D. J., Maisiak, R., Brown, S., and Koplan, A., "Acceptance by arthritis patients of clinical inquiry into their sexual adjustment." *Psychosomatics.* 27(8), pp. 576–579, 1986.

Blake, D. J., Maisiak, R., Holley, H. L., and Brown, S., "Sexual quality-of-life of patients with arthritis compared to arthritis-free controls." *Journal of Rheumatology.* 14(3), pp. 570–576, 1987.

Blake, D. J., Maisiak, R., Koplan, A. Alarcon, G. S., and Brown, S., "Sexual dysfunction among patients with arthritis." *Clinical Rheumatology.* 7(1), pp. 50–60, 1988.

Brassell, M. P., and Katz, W. A., "Sexuality and arthritis." In Katz, W. A. (ed.). *Diagnosis and Management of Rheumatic Diseases.* Philadelphia: Lippincott, 1988.

Buckwalter, K. C., Wernimont, T., and Buckwalter, J. A., "Musculo-skeletal conditions and sexuality II." *Sexuality and Disability.* 5(4), pp. 195–207, 1982.

Ehrlich, G. E., "Sexual problems of the arthritic." In Comfort, A. (ed.), *Sexual Consequences of Disability.* Philadelphia: G. F. Stickley, 1978.

Elst, P., Sybesma, T., van der Stadt, R. J., Prins, A. P. A., Muller, W. H., and den Butter, A., "Sexual problems in rheumatoid arthritis and ankylosing spondylitis." *Arthritis and Rheumatism.* 27, pp. 217–220, 1984.

Ferguson, K., and Figley, B., "Sexuality and rheumatic disease: A prospective study." *Sexuality and Disability.* 2, pp. 130–138, 1979.

Fisher, B., and Galler, R., "Friendship and fairness: How disability affects friendship between women." In Fine, M. and Asch, A. (eds.), *Women with Disabilities: Essays in Psychology, Politics, and Culture.* Philadelphia: Temple University Press, pp. 172–194, 1988.

Goleman, D., and Gurin, J. (eds.), *Mind Body Medicine: How to Use Your Mind for Better Health.* Yonkers, New York: Consumer Reports Books, 1993.

Halstead, L. S., "Sexual adjustment for arthritic patients." In Comfort, A. (ed.), *Sexual Consequences of Disability.* Philadelphia: G. F. Stickley, 1978.

Herstein, A., Hill, R. H., and Walters, K., "Adult sexuality and juvenile rheumatoid arthritis." *Journal of Rheumatology.* 4, pp. 35–39, 1977.

Hill, R. H., Herstien, A., and Walters, K., "Juvenile rheumatoid arthritis: Follow-up into adulthood: Medical, sexual and social status." *Canadian Medical Association Journal.* 114, pp. 790–794, 1976.

Kraaimaat, F. W., Bakker, A. H., Janssen, E., and Bijlsma, J. W. J., "Intrusiveness of rheumatoid arthritis on sexuality in male and female patients living with a spouse." *Arthritis Care and Research.* 9, pp. 120–125, 1996.

Kraaimaat, F. W., Van Dam-Baggen, C. M. J., and Bijlsma, J. W. J., "Associa-
    tion of social support and the spouse's reaction with psychological dis-
    tress in male and female patients with rheumatoid arthritis." *Journal of
    Rheumatology.* 22(4), pp. 644–648, 1995.

Kraaimaat, F. W., Van Dam-Baggen, C. M. J., and Bijlsma, J. W. J., "Depres-
    sion, anxiety and social support in rheumatoid arthritic women with-
    out and with a spouse." *Psychology and Health.* 10(5), pp. 387–396, 1995.

Lanza A. F., and Revenson, T. A., "Social support interventions for rheuma-
    toid arhritis patients: The cart before the horse?" *Health Education
    Quarterly.* 20, pp. 97–117, 1993.

Manne, S., and Zautra, A. J., "Spouse criticism and support: Their associa-
    tion with coping and psychological adjustment among women with
    rheumatoid arthritis." *Journal of Personality and Social Psychology.*
    56(4), pp. 608–617, 1989.

Manne, S., and Zautra, A. J., "Couples coping with chronic illness: Women
    with rheumatoid arthritis and their healthy husbands." *Journal of Be-
    havioral Medicine.* 13, pp. 327–342, 1990.

Melamed, B. G., and Brenner, G. F., "Social support and chronic medical
    stress: An interaction-based approach." *Journal of Social and Clinical
    Psychology.* 9, pp. 104–117, 1989.

Reich, J. W., and Zautra, A. J., "Spouse encouragement of self-reliance and
    other-reliance in rheumatoid arthritis couples." *Journal of Behavioral
    Medicine.* 18(3), pp. 249–260, 1995.

Revenson, T. A., and Majerovitz, S., "Spouses' support provision to chroni-
    cally ill patients." *Journal of Social and Personal Relationships.* 7(4), pp.
    575–586, 1990.

Revenson, T. A., and Majerovitz, S. D., "The effects of chronic illness on the
    spouse: Social resources as stress buffers." *Arthritis Care and Research.*
    4, pp. 63–72. 1991.

Richards, J., "Sex and arthritis." *Sexuality and Disability.* 3(2), pp. 97–104,
    1980.

Rowat, K. M., and Knafl, K. A., "Living with chronic pain: The spouse's per-
    spective." *Pain.* 23, pp. 259–271, 1985.

Schiaffine, K. M., and Revenson, T. A., "Relative contributions of spousal
    support and illness appraisals to depressed mood in arthritis patients."
    Arthritis Care and Research. 8(2), pp. 80–87, 1995.

Sipski, M. L., Craig, E. J., and Alexander, E. (Eds.), *Sexual Function in People
    with Disability and Chronic Illness: A Health Professional's Guide.*
    Gaithersburg, MD: Aspen Publishers, 1997.

Todd, R. C., Lightowler, C. D., and Harris, J., "Low friction arthroplasty of
    the hip joint and sexual activity." *Acta Orthopaedica Scandinavica.*
    44(6) pp. 690–693, 1973.

Tucker, J. S., Winkelman, D. K., Katz, J. N., and Bermas, B. L., "Ambivalence over emotional expression and psychological well-being among rheumatoid arthritis patients and their spouses." *Journal of Applied Social Psychology.* 29(2), pp. 271–290, 1999.

Turk, D. C., Flor, H., and Rudy, T. E., "Pain and families: I. Etiology, maintenance and psychosocial impact." *Pain.* 30, pp. 3–27, 1987.

Walsh, J. D., Blanchard, E. B., Kremer, J. M., and Blanchard, C. G., "The psychosocial effects of rheumatoid arthritis on the patient and the well partner." *Behaviour Research and Therapy.* 37(3), pp. 259–71, 1999.

Waltz, M., Kriegel, W., and van't Pad Bosch, P., "The social environment and health in rheumatoid arthritis: Marital quality predicts individual variability in pain severity." *Arthritis Care and Research.* 11(5), pp. 356–374, 1998.

Williamson, D., Robinson, M. E., and Melamed, B., "Pain behavior, spouse responsiveness, and marital satisfaction in patients with rheumatoid arthritis." *Behavior Modification.* 21(1), pp. 97–118, 1997.

Yoshino, S., and Uchida, S., "Sexual problems of women with rheumatoid arthritis." *Archives of Physical Medicine and Rehabilitation.* 62, pp. 122–123, 1981.

Zautra, A. J., Hoffman, J. M., Matt, K. S., Yocum, D., Potter, P. T., Castro W. L., and Roth, S., "An examination of individual differences in the relationship between interpersonal stress and disease activity among women with rheumatoid arthritis." *Arthritis Care and Research.* 11(4), pp. 271–279, 1998.

CHAPTER 9

1.   Reisine, S. T., Goodenow, C., & Grady, K. E., "The impact of rheumatoid arthritis on the homemaker." *Social Science and Medicine.* 25, pp. 89–95, 1987.

2.   Dura, J. R, and Beck, S. J., "A comparison of family functioning when mothers have chronic pain." *Pain.* 35(Oct., 1), pp. 79–89, 1988.

3.   Sloman, H., and Reilly, S., "Parenting with a disability: The issues." *Rehab and Community Care Management,* Spring 1998.

Bibliography

Arthritis Foundation, "Arthritis. The family. Making the difference." Brochure, 1987.

Arthritis Foundation, "Arthritis. Travel tips for people with arthritis." Brochure, 1988.

Arthritis Foundation, "Managing your activities." Brochure, 1997.

The Arthritis Society of Canada, BC and Yukon Division, "Tips for gardening with arthritis," undated.

Arthritis Foundation, "Arthritis on the job: You can work with it." Brochure, 1994.

Badley, E. M., "The impact of disabling arthritis." *Arthritis Care and Research.* 8, pp. 242–250, 1995.

Cyr, L., Occupational Therapist, Personal Interview, Vancouver, Canada, June 10, 1999.

Katz, P. P., "The impact of rheumatoid arthritis on life activites." *Arthritis Care and Research.* 8(Dec., 4), pp. 272–278, 1995.

Lorig, K., and Fries, J. F., *The Arthritis Helpbook, Fourth Edition.* Redding, Mass: Addison-Wesley Publishing Company, 1995.

Sliwa, J. L. "Occupational therapy assessment and management." In *Rehabilitation of Rheumatic Conditions,* by Ehrlich, George E, 1986.

CHAPTER 10

1. Ballard, W. T., and Buckwalter, W. T., "Operative treatment of rheumatic disease." *Primer on Rheumatic Disease.* 11, p. 443, 1997.

2. Wymenga, A. B., Horn. J. R., Theeuwes, A., Muytjens, H. L., and Slooff T. J., "Perioperative factors associated with septic arthritis after arthroplasty: prospective multicenter study of 362 knee and 2,651 hip operations." *Acta Orthopedica Scandanavia.* 63, pp. 665–671, 1992.

3. Adapted from *Surgery & Arthritis: What You Need to Know.* Atlanta, GA: The Arthritis Foundation, 1998.

4. *Surgery & Arthritis: What You Need to Know.* Atlanta, GA: The Arthritis Foundation, 1998.

5. Charnley, J., "Arthroplasty of the hip: A new operation." *The Lancet.* 1, p. 1129, 1961.

6. Cornell, C. N., and Ranawat, C. S., "The impact of modern cement techniques on acetabular fixation in cemented total hip replacement." *Journal of Arthroplasty.* 1, p. 197, 1986.

7. Galante, J. O., "Clinical results with the HGP cement less total hip prosthesis." In *Non-cemented Total Hip Arthroplast.* Fitzgerald, R., Jr. (ed.), New York: Raven Press, 1988.

8. Wolfe, F., and Zwillich, S. H., "The long-term outcomes of rheumatoid arthritis: A 23–year prospective, longitudinal study of total joint replacement and its predictors in 1,600 patients with rheumatoid arthritis." *Arthritis and Rheumatism.* 41, p. 1072–1082, 1998.

9. Poss, R., Ewald, F. C., Thomas, W. H., et al., "Complications of total hip replacement arthroplasty in patients with rheumatoid arthritis." *Journal of Bone and Joint Surgery* (United States). 58, p. 1130–1133, 1976.

10. Rand, J. A., and Ilstrup, D. M., "Survivorship analysis of total knee arthroplasty: Cumulative rates of survival of 9200 total knee replacement arthroplasties." *Journal of Bone and Joint Surgery* (United States). 73, p. 397, 1991.

11. Brady, O. H., Masri, B. A., Garbuz, D. S., and Duncan, C. P., "Joint re-

placement of the hip and knee—when to refer and what to expect."
Canadian Medical Association Journal. 163(10), p. 1285–1291, 2000.

CHAPTER 11

1. Nelson, JL. and Ostensen, M., "Pregnancy and Rheumatoid Arthritis,"
    Rheumatic Disease Clinics of North America. 23: 195–212, 1997.
2. Spector, TD., Roman, E., and Silman, AJ., "The pill, parity, and rheuma-
    toid arthritis," *Arthritis and Rheumatism*, 33 (6), 782–789, 1990.
3. Hannaford, PC., Kay, CR., and Hirsch, S. "Oral contraceptives and
    rheumatoid arthritis: New data from the Royal College of General
    Practitioners' oral contraception study." *Annals of the Rheumatic Dis-
    eases*, 49, 744–746, 1990.
4. Nelson, and Ostensen, 1997.
5. Nelson and Ostensen, 1997.
6. Van der Horst-Bruinsma, I.E., de Vries, R.R.P., de Buck, P.D.M., van
    Schendel, P. W., Breedveld, F. C., Schreuder, G. M., and Hazes, J. M. W.
    "Influence of HLA-class II incompatibility between mother and fetus
    on the development and course of rheumatoid arthritis of the mother."
    Annals of the Rheumatic Diseases, 57, 28–290, 1998.
7. Nelson and Ostensen, 1997.
8. Nelson and Ostensen, 1997.
9. Nelson and Ostensen, 1997.
10. Ramsey-Goldman, R. and Schilling, E. "Immunosuppressive drug use
    during pregnancy." *Rheumatic Disease Clinics of North America*, 23 (1),
    149–167, 1997.
11. Ostensen, M., "Optimisation of antirheumatic drug treatment in preg-
    nancy." *Clinical Pharmacokinetics*, 27 (6), 486–503, 1994.
12. McKenry, L.M. and Salerno, E., *Mosby's Pharmacology in Nursing.* St.
    Louis: Harcourt Health Sciences, 2000.
13. Ostensen, M. and Ostensen, H., "Safety of nonsteroidal anti-inflamma-
    tory drugs in pregnant patients with rheumatic disease." *Journal of
    Rheumatology*, 23 (6), 1045–1049, 1996.
14. Park-Wyllie, L., Mazzotta, P., Pastuszak, A. Moretti, M.E., Beique, L.,
    Hunnisett, L., et al. "Birth defects after maternal exposure to corticos-
    teroids: prospective cohort study and meta-analysis of epidemiological
    studies." *Teratology*, 62: pp. 385–392, 2000.
15. Ramsey-Goldman and Schilling, 1997.
16. Little, B.B., "Immunosuppressant therapy during gestation." *Seminars
    in Perinatology*, 21 (2), 143–148, 1997.
17. Rains, C.P., Noble, S., and Faulds, D., "Sulfasalazine: A review of its
    pharmacological properties and therapeutic efficacy in the treatment
    of rheumatoid arthritis." *Drugs*, 50 (1), 137–156, 1995.

18. Ostensen, 1994.

19. Mogadam, M., Dobbuis, W.O., Korelitz, B.I., et al. "Pregnancy in inflammatory bowel disease: Effect of sulfasalazine and corticosteriods on fetal outcome." *Gastroenterology*. Vol. 80, p. 72, 1981.

20. Fedorkow, D.M., Persaud, D., Nimrod, C.A., "Inflammatory bowel disease: A controlled study of late pregnancy outcome." *American Journal of Obstetrics and Gynecology*, Vol. 160, 998, 1989.

21. Azad Khan, A.Z., TruHou S.C., Placental and mammary disposition of sulfasalazine," *British Medical Journal*. Vol. 2, pg. 1553, 1972.

22. Nelson and Ostensen, 1997.

23. Ostensen, 1994.

24. Little, 1997.

25. Buckley, L.M., Bullaboy, C.A., Leichtman, L., Marquez, M., "Multiple congenital anomalies associated with weekly low-dose methotrexate treatment of the mother." *Arthritis and Rheumatism*, 40 (5), 971–973, 1997.

26. Nelson and Ostensen, 1997.

27. Ramsey-Goldman and Schilling, 1997.

28. Ramsey-Goldman and Schilling, 1997.

29. Little, 1997.

30. Ostensen, 1994

31. Ramsey-Goldman and Schilling, 1997.

32. Ramsey-Goldman and Schilling, 1997.

33. Ramsey-Goldman and Schilling, 1997.

34. Ramsey-Goldman and Schilling, 1997.

35. Momohara, S., and Aritomi, H., "Osteoporosis in collegen diseases," *Japanese Journal of Clinical Medicine*, 52, 2420–2425, 1994.

36. Hall, G.M., Spector, T. D., Griffin, AJ., Jawad, A.S., Hall, M.L., and Doyle, D.V., "The effect of rheumatoid arthritis and steroid therapy on bone density in postmenopausal women." *Arthritis and Rheumatism*, 36, 1510–1516, 1993.

37. Butler, R.C., Davie, M.W., Worsfold, M., and Sharp, C.A., "Bone mineral content in patients with rheumatoid arthritis: Relationship to low-dose steroid therapy." *British Journal of Rheumatology*, 30, 86–90, 1991.

38. Kreoger, H., Honkanen, R., Saarikoski, S., and Alhava, E., "Decreased axial bone mineral density in perimenopausal women with rheumatoid arthritis—a population based study." *Annals of the Rheumatic Diseases*, 53, 18–23, 1994.

39. Leboff, M.S., Wade, J.P., Mackowiak, S., el-Hajj Fuleihan, G., Zangari, M., and Liang, M.H. "Low dose prednisone does not affect calcium homeostasis or bone density in postmenopausal women with rheumatoid arthirits." *Journal of Rheumatology*, 18, 339–344, 1991.

40. Lichtman, R. "Perimenopausal and postmenopausal hormone replace-

ment therapy, part 1: An update of the literature on benefits and risks." *Journal of Nurse-Midwifery*, 41, 3–28, 1996.

41. Silman, A., and Hochberg, M. C., *Epidemiology of the Rheumatic Diseases*. Oxford: Oxford University Press, 1993.

42. Jorgensen, C., Picot, M.C., Bologna, C., and Sany, J., "Oral contraception, parity, breastfeeding, and severity of rheumatoid arthritis." *Annals of the Rheumatic Diseases*, 55 (2), 94–98, 1996.

43. Spector, T.D., Roman, E., and Silman, A.J., "The pill, parity, and rheumatoid arthritis." *Arthritis and Rheumatism*, 33 (6), 782–789, 1990.

44 Nelson and Ostensen, 1997.

45. Silman, 1998.

46. Hannaford, Kay, and Hirsch, 1990.

47. Silman, A., Kay, A., and Brennan, P., "Timing of pregnancy in relation to the onset of rheumatoid arthritis." *Arthritis and Rheumatism*, 35 (2), 152–155., 1992.

48. Silman, 1998.

49. Van der Horst-Bruinsma, I.E., de Vries, R. R. P., de Buck, P.D.M., van Schendel, PW., Breedveld, F.C., Schreuder, G. M., and Hazes, J.M.W., "Influence of HLA-class II incompatibility between mother and fetus on the development and course of rheumatoid arthritis of the mother." *Annals of the Rheumatic Diseases*, 57, 286–290, 1998.

50. Nelson and Ostensen, 1997.

51. Gilbert, C., "Neurotransmitter status and remission of rheumatoid arthritis in pregnancy." *Journal of Rheumatology*, 21 (6), 1056–1060, 1994.

52. Van der Horst-Bruinsma, de Vries, de Buck, van Schendel, Breedveld, Schreuder and Hazes, 1998.

53. Nelson and Ostensen, 1997.

54. Ostensen, M., and Nelson, J.L., "Bits and pieces in a puzzle—Rheumatoid arthritis and pregnancy." *British Journal of Rheumatology*, 34, 1–7, 1995.

55. Silman, 1998.

56. Nelson, Voigt, Koepsell, Dugowson, and Daling, 1992.

57. Hannaford, Kay, and Hirsch, 1990.

58. Silman, Kay, and Brennan, 1992.

59. Silman and Hochberg, 1993.